It's okay
to hate
this guide.

You can
still use it.

To all the worried, wired and overworked, the stress-heads, jitterbugs and anxious wrecks, this is for you.

BLOOMSBURY PUBLISHING
Bloomsbury Publishing Plc
50 Bedford Square, London, WC1B 3DP, UK

BLOOMSBURY, BLOOMSBURY
PUBLISHING and the Diana logo are
trademarks of Bloomsbury Publishing Plc

First published in Great Britain 2020

ISBN: HB: 9-781-5266-2843-5
eBook: 9-781-5266-2844-2

10 9 8 7 6 5 4 3 2 1

Editor: Xa Shaw Stewart
Project Editor: Sophie Elletson
Designer: Emily Voller
Illustrator: Elisa Cunningham

The publishers would like to thank
Megan Macadam for her guidance on the
mental health issues that are covered
within this book

The stretches and exercise guidance on pages
104 to 105 are featured with kind permission
from Kit Laughlin

Printed and bound in China by Toppan
Leefung Printing

Bloomsbury Publishing Plc makes every
effort to ensure that the papers used in
the manufacture of our books are natural,
recyclable products made from wood grown
in well-managed forests. Our manufacturing
processes conform to the environmental
regulations of the country of origin

To find out more about our authors and books visit
www.bloomsbury.com and sign up for our newsletters

# Burnout Survival Kit

BLOOMSBURY PUBLISHING
LONDON · OXFORD · NEW YORK · NEW DELHI · SYDNEY

# SO YOU'RE BURNING OUT?

Your body aches. Your brain feels like a mouldy wrung-out dishcloth. You can barely get anything done and, hang on, why are you even doing this job anyway? Is there something wrong with you? Nope. You're just burning out.

Welcome. You've found the right book.

According to the Government's Health and Safety Executive, one in five Brits suffer workplace stress and half a million of us are stressed to the point of illness. Things are so bad the World Health Organisation has reclassified burnout as an occupational condition. And if you throw in stagnant wages, unhealthy workplaces, poor management, awkward work relationships and the sinking feeling that you're doing the wrong thing with your life? Then you've all got the ingredients for total burnout.

Which is why I wrote this book. After a stint in advertising, I became a freelance screenwriter. And I thought it was fabulous. I ate nothing but chocolate, never took breaks, worked in my jammies, and became obsessed with 'making it'. Until I was having chest pains and breathing problems and struggling just to get out of bed. I thought I was having a heart attack. Turns out it was just some big ol' scoops of stress, anxiety and depression all rolled into one nightmare burnout sundae. Delicious.

*Burnout Survival Kit* is the book I wish I'd had before – practical suggestions to help you through when things are *already bad*. There's no mystical magic about unleashing your inner corporate superhero, no weird productivity diagrams, and certainly no nonsense about working 'smarter'. The advice in here may not cure burnout completely, but it does offer instant relief. So whether you're just starting to sizzle or fully scorched to a crisp, breathe out. You've got a Burnout Survival Kit.

Imogen

# CONTENTS

# LONG-TERM PROBLEMS

## READING LIST

## ENDNOTES

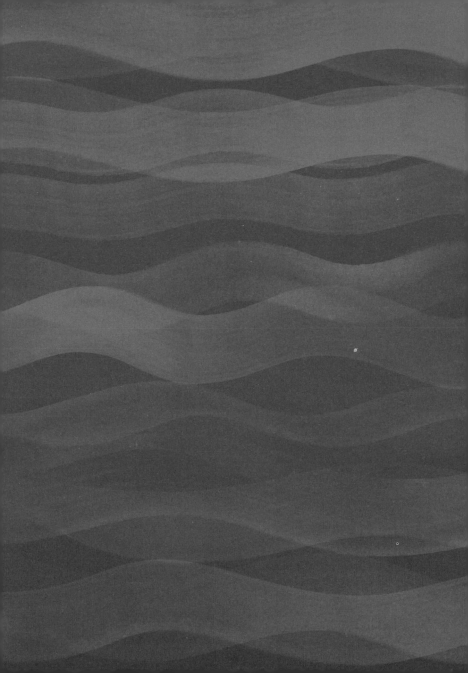

# EMERGENCY PROBLEMS

# I'M HAVING A PANIC ATTACK

Racing heartbeat

Hot flushes

Ringing in your ears

Feeling faint

Chills

Feeling of dread or fear of dying

Sweating

Shaky limbs

Nausea

Choking sensation

Churning stomach

Chest pain

Dizziness

Shortness of breath

Numbness or pins and needles

Tingling sensation in your fingers

Dry mouth

Trembling

Needing to go to the toilet

Feeling disconnected from your body

### You are not dying.

Your body is producing some pretty bog-standard anxiety sensations, but your brain has decided they herald the end of the world. These sensations will end and you will be okay, even if your brain is trying to tell you otherwise.

### Use coping statements.

Repeat to yourself that you will be fine, you can get through this, it will last only 20 to 30 minutes – and often much less than that.

### Do breathing exercises.

Breathe in as slowly and as deeply as you can, in through your nose and out through your mouth. I find it helps to place a hand on my stomach to ensure I am breathing right into my belly. (This is called diaphragmatic breathing.) If your breath is shallow, rapid or gulping, or you can't stop thinking about your breathing, you are probably hyperventilating, which means you are breathing out too much carbon dioxide. Breathe into a clean paper bag to help normalise the oxygen levels in your body.

### Ground yourself.

There are two great ways to do this. The first is to close your eyes and focus your awareness on your body. Start by relaxing your toes, then your feet, and work your way right up to your head. Don't forget all the little muscles in your face, like your jaw and brow.

The second is called the 5-4-3-2-1 technique and it works by helping you focus on the world around you. Notice five things you can see, four things you can touch, three things you can hear, two things you can smell, and one thing you can taste.

### Inhale a special smell.

I know it seems like the comedy of a highly strung rich woman reaching for her smelling salts, but I've found it immensely useful to carry a small vial of rosemary and mint essential oils mixed together. For me, inhaling this scent triggers my deep breathing and has become linked to memories of relaxation. I also dab it on my temples and between my eyebrows if I feel anxious. There might be a lovely scent that works for you!

## Once the attack has passed, take time to lower your stress levels.

Make a cup of aromatic tea. Take a bath. Cuddle a pet. Play a chilled-out video game like Animal Crossing, Kind Words, Journey, Coffee Talk or Monument Valley. Take a nap. If the weather is nice, a gentle walk is a great way to calm yourself and return your breathing to normal.

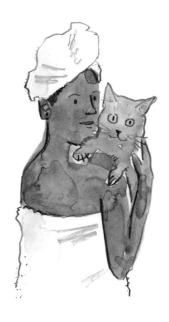

## Release tight areas in your body.

Do you know where your body stores stress? It took me a long time to realise I clench my jaw, purse my lips and tense my hips – almost every single day. Other common places of tension are the brow, neck, shoulders, tummy, hands and feet.

It's useful to stretch regularly, making sure you 'breathe into the stretch'. This means using your new diaphragmatic breaths to increase blood flow to your muscles and stop your nervous system hitting the emergency brakes on your movement. To get started, I recommend Kit Laughlin's Daily Five stretches (see pages 103–105), yoga or sports massage. You might also like stretching on a foam roller or with a lacrosse or tennis ball for 'trigger point' release.

## Manage your cortisol.

Spikes and crashes in your blood sugar levels can hugely affect your mood. That's because sugar causes your adrenal glands to release cortisol, which is the same hormone that is released when you are stressed. Try to keep your blood sugar levels under control by minimising sweet foods, smoking, caffeine, alcohol and heavily processed foods.

## Get better sleep.

Most of us need seven to nine hours of sleep each night. Unfortunately, if you struggle with anxiety, you may also have inherited its fun little buddy, insomnia. So take the time to make your bed cosy. You need a space that is comfortable, quiet, dark and cool. Specifically, between 15 and 23°C[1]. If you haven't already, invest in a quality mattress, nice breathable sheets and a supportive pillow.

Now that your bed's all snug, you need to work on the vibes. Ban yourself from working or doing anything stressful in bed. You want your brain to build a strong association between lying in bed and feeling relaxed or sleepy. It can also help to design a wind-down routine – taking a shower, sipping herbal tea, popping on a face mask – which signals to your brain that it's time to get your sleep on. Lying in bed is also a great place to practise your diaphragmatic breathing and grounding exercises.

You can help yourself during the day, too. Exercising is a brilliant way to reduce stress and help tire yourself out a bit. Try to avoid caffeine after 2pm and heavy foods at least three hours before you go to bed. And be sure to avoid bright screens at least an hour before bedtime[2].

If you still aren't sleeping well, it's worth speaking to your GP about the strategies and medications that might work for you.

# I FEEL MISERABLE AND I DON'T KNOW WHY

Okay, first things first:

- When did you last drink water?

- When did you last eat a healthy meal?

- When did you last get outside?

- When did you last exercise or stretch?

- When did you last bathe?

- When did you last get a good night's sleep?

If you just nodded through that list thinking, 'Yeah, whatever, let's skip to the good stuff,' then you can stop right now, thank you very much! Read the list again, look in the mirror, and tell yourself you're taking good care of your body.

Because I know you've been sat hunched over for hours, slurping coffee, grinding your jaw, neurotically checking your social media and wondering why you feel so queasy. I know this because I do it, too. And to be honest, it's a bit like dumping all your garbage in the garden and wondering why the flowers won't grow.

Give your body a chance to be happy. Get at least four items checked off the list before you try other strategies because, chances are, some of those weird jittery feelings? That's your body crying out for a little R.E.S.P.E.C.T.

## Cry it out.

Find yourself a comfortable place to just let it all out. Maybe that's the shower. Maybe that's your bed. Maybe that's in front of the new season of *Queer Eye*. Whatever it takes, give yourself permission to release that bad energy.

## Take a useful break.

You may have been staring at your screen for hours, days or even weeks without getting any good work done, and you read 'take a break' and think, 'Pfft, I wish!' But at this point you need more than a break. You need to completely reset your mind. Whether you're freelance or full-time, take a mental-health day. Go on a long walk. Take a train out of town. Try tai chi, dance or Pilates. Call a friend. Book a massage. Clean and reorganise a space. Stretch. Decompress.

If you really can't take a day off, you still need time away from your workspace. Use your lunch break to get outside and walk. If you can, spend the rest of your day working from a local café or library. At the very least, work on something else.

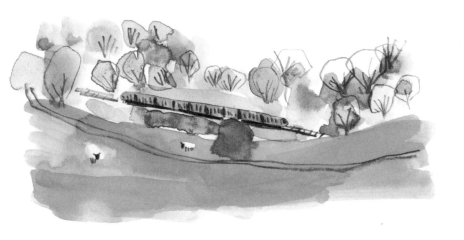

# PERMISSION SLIPS

To not be helpful today

To drink wine in the bath

To not take that advice

To watch trashy telly

To be alone

To ask a friend for a hug

To make bad art

To not reassure everyone you're okay

To pick or buy yourself flowers

To ask someone to do something for you

To eat carbs

To do nothing productive whatsoever

To wrap yourself in a duvet burrito

To switch off your phone

To take a day off work

To not explain racism/sexism/your expertise to that person

To not smile at strangers

To cancel your plans

## Turn your worries into a checklist.

If you have too many thoughts swirling around your head, it's difficult to concentrate, let alone get work done. Let each worry surface and jot them down – even if they're little things like 'I have a headache' or 'I forgot it's my mate's birthday' or 'I still haven't donated that clothing I left in a pile on the floor.' Pick one or two you can commit to solving by the end of the day.

If you've jotted down some things that can't be easily solved, like 'I just feel upset,' designate some 'worry time' for the day. This cognitive behavioural therapy technique gives you a specific time and place just to worry, which helps stop your worries interrupting the rest of your day.

## You may have a problem with your approach.

It may be that there is something fundamentally 'not right' about the way you are going about this work. If it's making you miserable and you don't know why, it's time to seek feedback and a fresh perspective. This doesn't necessarily need to be your boss or your client, but whomever you ask, make sure you listen to everything they say with an open mind. Don't let yourself immediately come up with objections, even if their suggestions are strange or irritating. The point is to locate the problem area so you can fix it, not defend it to death just to make yourself feel slightly better.

## Ask Spock.

If you've never seen any *Star Trek*, don't panic. All you need to know is that Spock is a half-alien who lives by pure logic and reason with as little interference from emotion as possible. Now, imagine Spock sitting next to you. (That's it. Use your imagination for good instead of worry!) Explain what's rattling around in your head and see what he says. Chances are, he'll give you the straight-talking advice you kind of knew would help but were refusing to take. I tend to find myself saying, 'Spock! I left an email for way too long and now I'm embarrassed to reply!' He says, 'Have you considered just sending the email?'

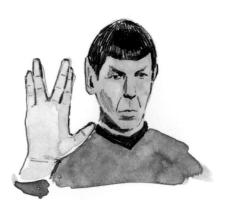

## You may be depressed or anxious.

Most people have bad days or a bad week, but it may be time to seek professional help if you feel persistently sad or worried for weeks or months.

I understand the feelings of shame, defeat and fear associated with this. I have been there. I cried the first few times I searched online for a counsellor. Even when I finally booked in, I nearly didn't go.

But if I can do it, you can! I mean, I sobbed. *Every time*. But in the end, it was a huge relief to externalise fears and start to feel okay about them. And although it didn't happen immediately, after a while I noticed I had developed stronger empathy – not just for others, but for myself as well.

If I can offer any advice from this experience, it's that seeking help and accessing NHS services isn't always easy, so don't take it personally. There'll probably be some confusing form to fill out or a grumpy receptionist who says there are no appointments for ages, so make sure you don't interpret this as a sign that you don't need or deserve help. You do. Everybody deserves to be happy and healthy at work.

# I'M HAVING DARK THOUGHTS

No dream is worth sacrificing your health and happiness. Do not accept the myth that successful people must be exhausted tortured souls in order to be authentic. You are worthy. You deserve to be happy. And you are not your career. You are a beautiful person enriching this world, just by being here and being yourself. I love you.

### Just focus on getting through today.

Try not to think about the future, just do whatever you need to do to get through the day. Cancel your commitments. Be kind to yourself.

### Stay away from drugs and alcohol.

Yes, any type of drug and any type of alcohol.

## Do something you usually enjoy.

Spend some time with a pet. Make your favourite food or try a new recipe. Take a long shower and really scrub yourself clean. Wear your favourite outfit. Watch uplifting movies or TV shows. Spend the day snuggled in bed, armed with your favourite book and some delicious snacks. Play a video game. Do a crossword. Try making or fixing something. Let yourself scream, cry, stamp and sigh. Do a kindness for someone else or the environment. Read a gentle self-help book.* Meditate. This too shall pass.

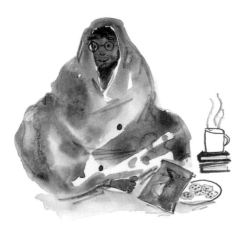

* I know hanging around the self-help book section feels a bit like wearing a sign around your neck that says 'I'm sad!' but there are people out there who are waiting to connect with you on all this tricky, icky stuff. I absolutely love *How to Survive the End of the World (When It's In Your Own Head)* by Aaron Gillies and *Reasons to Stay Alive* by Matt Haig.

## Get yourself to a safe place.

Going to a friend's or family member's place is a great way to ensure your own safety and to share the burden of your thoughts with another trusted soul. Even if it's someone you haven't spoken to in a long time, reach out anyway. People understand.

## Be around other people.

You don't have to talk about yourself if you don't want to. Let them talk to you.

## Find yourself some long-term support.

If you regularly return to thoughts about suicide or harming yourself, it's time to install some much stronger support. Book in with your GP today to discuss your options, such as professional therapy. There are wonderful people out there who have dedicated their lives to helping people through this. Let them support you, too.

## Contact a helpline.

If you can't stop yourself thinking about dark things, contact a helpline now. See the opposite page for some friendly UK options, or search the net.

# Help is Always Available

**Samaritans**
116 113
jo@samaritans.org

**Shout (if you prefer texting)**
Text SHOUT to 85258

**Papyrus (for under 35s)**
0800 068 41 41
pat@papyrus-uk.org

**Campaign Against Living Miserably (for men)**
0800 58 58 58

**Mind (mental health resources)**
mind.org.uk

**NHS Urgent Mental Health Helplines**
nhs.uk/service-search/mental-health/find-
an-urgent-mental-health-helpline

**If you have harmed yourself, call**
999

# SHORT-TERM PROBLEMS

'Each person deserves a day away in which no problems are confronted, no solutions searched for. Each of us needs to withdraw from the cares which will not withdraw from us.'

MAYA ANGELOU

# I FEEL SICK WITH STRESS

| | | |
|---|---|---|
| Headaches | Chest pain | Shallow breathing or hyperventilating |
| Feeling sick, dizzy or faint | High blood pressure | Sexual problems |
| Muscle tension or pain | | Difficulty sleeping |
| Stomach problems | Blurred eyesight or sore eyes | Having nightmares |
| Indigestion or heartburn | Grinding your teeth | Feeling snappy or irritable |
| Constipation or diarrhoea | Clenching your jaw | Feeling tired all the time |

It's okay to feel stressed at work. We all do! Sometimes it can even be motivating. But there's a big difference between the occasional spike and an endless high-velocity nightmare. That's because when your brain detects a stressful situation (lions! Tigers! That work is due *tomorrow*!), it leads to the release of a hormone called cortisol. This primes your body for instant action, which is really rather handy – if you're trying to run from lions and tigers. Not so handy for almost everything else.

Experiencing high levels of cortisol for long periods of time wreaks havoc on your brain[3], which can physically shrink and lose connections in the bit that deals with your decision-making, concentration, judgement and social interaction. Signals also decrease in the hippocampus – the region that handles your learning, memories and stress control[4]. So, yep. The more stressed you are, the worse you are at controlling it.

Forgive yourself for feeling a little crazy, and let's see what we can do about it.

## Take stress seriously.

These are not symptoms that will resolve themselves if you just work 'smarter' – whatever that is. Even if taking the time to deal with stress seems like the most stressful thing you could do right now, in the long run it could change your life. If you try a few strategies and nothing helps, it's time to book in with your GP.

In 2019, the UK lost 12.8 million working days to work-related stress, depression and anxiety[5].

## It's okay to say no.

Nobody is going to think less of you. Admitting when your plate is full is a sign of emotional maturity. If you're always being asked to squeeze in 'urgent' work, don't just cram it on top of everything else. Ask what will be delayed or sacrificed to make room for it.

If you work alone and you're constantly saying yes to everything, then you need to have a stern word with the boss. (That's you!)

# The
# Thing
# About
# <u>Yoga</u>

Okay, I get it: *everyone* recommends yoga and *everyone* sounds utterly insane when they do it. 'It's pure bliss,' they gush, with their glassy, cult-like eyes. 'You haven't lived until you've done a lotus headstand variation!' But the thing is, yoga doesn't work because you've learned to contort yourself into a pretzel. Don't even begin to give a toss about that. Yoga works because it's an easy guided entry to diaphragmatic breathing.

If you do give yoga a chance, focus on your breath. Deep breathing is one of the best ways to cope with stress and anxiety. Of course, there are other entries into breathing practice, but doing a yoga session really forces you to stick at it for 30 minutes or more. Plus, there's something to be said for an ancient Indian art that has been popular since the fifth century BCE.

## Breathe like a yogi.

Even if you're feeling less yogi and more Yogi Bear (plump, hairy, motivated solely by snacks), deep breathing is a powerful tool when it comes to stress. And I get it. It sounds so simple it's almost insulting. But numerous studies have found that deep breathing induces a state of tranquillity[6]. The best part is, you can get started right now. You read that right. Place one hand on your belly and one hand on your heart, then breathe in through your nose and deeply into your belly for five full seconds. Then exhale slowly through your mouth for another five full seconds.

Try ten breaths this way, while dropping your gaze or closing your eyes to gain awareness of any tension in your body. Trust me, the more you practise this, the more it becomes a kind of Pavlovian reflex for chilling the hell out. If you'd like more of a guided experience, try the NHS Stress and Anxiety Companion app or the Pacifica app.

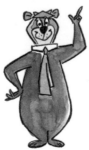

## Try a mood journal.

Tracking your moods and symptoms each day can be incredibly revealing. Maybe you have specific triggers, like deadlines or public speaking. Or maybe you're more of a hot-pot frog, suddenly hitting your limit when you've taken on too much. Developing self-awareness through journaling is a great way to anticipate the things that will stress you out, so you can prepare accordingly. (Plus, it's a fantastic excuse for new stationery!) If you're more technologically minded, there are some helpful mood-tracking apps out there, like Daylio, or Flo for women.

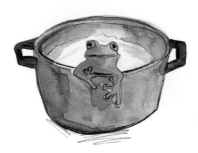

## Take control of your notifications.

Notifications are tiny little red stress demons, constantly tapping you on the shoulder and screaming HEY, THERE'S 50% OFF SOME PRODUCT YOU REGRET BUYING THREE YEARS AGO! You do not need this. Nobody needs this. Especially when you're so stressed.

In fact, checking emails *less* regularly is scientifically shown to reduce your stress[7]. So turn off all those automated notifications and choose your own timetable for actively checking messages. Maybe that's once per hour. Maybe that's as little as twice a day. You'll know what's right for you and your work. If you read this and think, 'Pfft, in my dreams!' then interrogate your reaction. Emails do not require split-second replies.

## Lean on your friends.

While having large numbers of Facebook friends increases your stress[8], a strong social circle in real life has a startlingly positive impact on your health and mortality[9]. In fact, one ten-minute chat with a friend boosts your problem-solving abilities[10]. But don't panic if it's hard for you to find friends as an adult. All you really need to do is let yourself become a familiar face where you work. Scientifically, the more people see you, the more they like you[11]. Try sticking to a simple routine, such as greeting colleagues every morning, going to the same coffee shop each afternoon, and joining an evening class.

## Can you reduce some physical symptoms?

If you're struggling to uncover the causes of your stress, try targeting some of its effects. Common side effects like lack of sleep, poor diet, poor hygiene or anaemia could be tackled while you work to understand your stress. It's also a great time to get serious about your addictions, like drinking, smoking and even social media.

## Learn how you like to relax.

I love it when I'm stressed and people tell me to 'just relax'. (Oh, *thank you*! If I had only *relaxed*, I wouldn't be in this mess!) The trick is to figure out the activities that make you feel relaxed, so you can pre-emptively build them into your schedule. In other words, rather than waiting until you hit crisis point, you'll have regular points of deliberate relaxation throughout your working week. These things can be physical, like running and dancing, or something creative, like colouring, pottery, painting, cooking and gardening.

Don't expect yourself to be good. At least not right away. Just because you're a grown-up doesn't mean everything you do needs to be professional. Are you being paid for this? No. Are you going to launch an Instagram career in pasta jewellery? Let's hope not. Lean into the freedom of being crap at something.

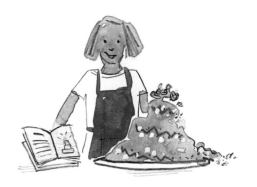

## Get a move on!

You knew this was coming. Exercise is a very well-documented stress reliever. The good news is you don't have to buy a load of ugly Lycra and utterly thrash yourself – unless you're into that. Turns out, *any* type of exercise will combat stress[12]. So why not do something you actually like? You could even learn a new skill, like the rumba. Imagine yourself at parties if you could rumba!

I sometimes trick myself by putting on a nice outfit to go for a long walk, or doing yoga at home in my pyjamas. It's worth noting, however, that stress impairs your efforts to be physically active[13], so go easy on yourself. It's not you, it's the stress. Start small and build up from there.

# I DREAD GOING TO WORK

Why is it that 7pm on a Sunday night feels like 11pm on any other night? Because Monday. Monday is coming. You struggle to wake up, you drag yourself into the shower, you barely get to work on time, you daydream about switching places with your cat... (Just me?)

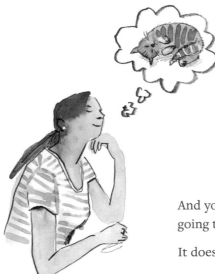

And you wonder, is it always going to feel like this?

It doesn't have to.

## Develop 'sustainable attitude'.

There is a lot of good in the phrase, 'Do what you love and you'll never work a day in your life!' But let's be real: it does come with a bit of a whiff. Because even the ultimate dream job requires you to do some crappy stuff you will simply never love. (Life as a cat, for example, comes with someone like me, desperately trying to touch your toe beans.) 'Sustainable attitude' is not about lowering your expectations. It's about forgiving yourself for not loving every single damn second of your work life. It's about being kind to yourself and others. And most importantly, it's about picking your battles.

## Take one day at a time.

Break your day into small chunks built around at least three tea breaks, two meal breaks and a wellness walk. Those are your rewards. Now make a list of the things you need to get done and identify which are the truly Cursed Jobs. For me, Cursed Jobs are the things I simply cannot stand doing, like booking dentist appointments, chasing invoices or reconciling my accounts. Do just one Cursed Job per day, as a treat.

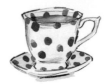

## Work out what is actually creating the dread.

Listen to the things you find yourself griping about. There is probably something to be done about most of them. If you're surrounded by people who moan about everything, try befriending a different group. If you feel underappreciated, bored and unchallenged, these are great reasons to have a discussion with your supervisor or rethink your career approach.

If you work for yourself, it's time to think about how you manage yourself. And if you feel like you just don't care about *anything*, you need to create reasons to care by writing or rewriting your life plan. This gives you perspective on all the irritating stuff, so you can see how it leads to the better stuff. (For more on motivation, flip to page 85, and to consider your career trajectory, try page 177.)

## Have a Happy Hour.

No, not that kind. Set aside one hour out of your day that is just for you. Even if it's at 10pm.

## Ask for better work to do.

Proactivity is never a bad look. Sometimes the best way to start doing work you actually enjoy is to put your hand up and ask for it. Identify the people around you whose careers you would like to emulate and find ways to offer them help, making it clear you'd love to follow in their footsteps. It sounds cheesy but showing someone that you admire their life choices is a great way to find a mentor.

You could also identify training or new qualifications, which your employer will probably pay for if you make a good case for it.

If you work alone, look around for little opportunities to push and inspire yourself, like competitions, grants or interesting workshops and talks.

## The grass may well be greener.

Consider launching a casual job search or looking into retraining options, just to see what is out there. If you start to feel inspired by what you find, start doing one thing per day to get yourself out of the situation that you're in. That could be anything from editing one section of your CV, to getting yourself a professional new haircut, to sparking a charming conversation with your boss in anticipation of getting a good recommendation.

# I'M OVERWHELMED BY MY WORKLOAD

There you were, feeling perfectly whelmed, when suddenly everything was all too much. You're panicking, you're running out of time and your to-do list is longer than a loo roll. And the worst part? Nobody has any sympathy for it. It's like we all think it's perfectly natural to feel tense, disoriented and completely swamped at work. So here's my radical suggestion: let's not.

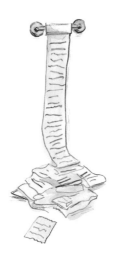

## Start with a list of what you're *not* going to work on.

This is a way of forgiving yourself for not being able to do every single little thing and focussing on what really requires your attention. Jot down all the stuff that needs doing but isn't right-this-second urgent. Now take a good look – and a deep breath. Everything on this list will get done, just not today. Put it somewhere safe and make a new list of the things you absolutely must do today – ideally no more than three. This is now *all* you need to think about.

## Ask for help prioritising your work.

Sometimes we feel so buried under our work it's impossible to see where to begin. In this case, the best thing to do is ask someone to decide for you. This could be a friend or a colleague, but it could also be the basis for a frank discussion with your manager or supervisor.

## Keep a 'blue head'.

This is a term the All Blacks rugby team uses to describe a free feeling of flow, where they acknowledge the pressure they are under while maintaining a cool, calm, clear-headed playing style. It's the opposite of what they call 'red head', which is feeling tight, inhibited, results-oriented, anxious, aggressive, overcompensating and desperate[14]. Essentially, this simple division is a great way to recognise when seemingly positive behaviours – wanting badly to succeed, pushing hard, considering minor details – only get in the way of your performance.

To get out of a red head and back into the blue, the All Blacks use deep deliberate breaths, then 'anchor' themselves with a physical reminder that brings them back to the present moment. (This could be stamping the earth or grabbing their wrist.) Finally, they repeat one of their mantras, such as 'Better people make better All Blacks.' Try coming up with your own blue-head mantra. I came up with 'Stop, breathe, write it down.'

## Tidy up a bit.

Working in a messy environment can increase stress and anxiety, and lead to emotional exhaustion[15]. Spend a few minutes on a quick cleaning blitz and you'll also clear out your head.

## It's okay to go slowly.

You simply cannot work at full speed, day after day after day. That'll get you nothing but a priority boarding pass for Burnout Airlines, destination Hell. Find a comfortable pace and stick to it.

## Avoid multi-tasking.

Multi-tasking is supposed to be something that smart, efficient people do, but it's actually a total time-waster. Switching between tasks creates little 'mental blocks' that can steal as much as 40% of your working time[16]. Multi-taskers also can't remember things as well as those who focus on one thing[17]. So if you find yourself trying to listen to a video conference while you type up notes, check emails and send emojis to your mates, stop! Ron Swanson says it best: 'Never half-ass two things. Whole-ass one thing.'

## Don't fall for performative busy-ness.

It can feel good to huff around the place, letting everyone know just how busy you are. But are you really that busy? Or do you just like people to think you're busy? Those who believe they work long hours tend to significantly overestimate the real time they spend working – and worse, if you say to yourself things like, 'I work 70 hours a week!' your brain reacts as if it's true[18]. In other words, constantly reminding yourself that you're overworked has a psychosomatic, self-fulfilling effect.

'If you hear a
voice within
you saying,
"You are not a
painter," then by
all means paint,
and that voice
will be silenced.'

VINCENT VAN GOGH

# I DON'T HAVE ENOUGH TIME TO FINISH THIS WORK

How does a workday seem to last forever and yet the amount of time you actually have feels like seven seconds? It is truly cruel sorcery and I can offer no explanation. Fortunately, I can offer a few tips on how to manage your time and get things done.

## Start with a 'Condor Moment'.

This British Army phrase refers to the brand of cigarettes once supplied to troops that the soldiers would often smoke before committing to an action. Thankfully, you don't need a smoking habit to take your own Condor Moment. Simply get up from your desk, breathe, make a cup of tea, and give yourself a minute to calm and order your thoughts. And then you can move on to fixing them.

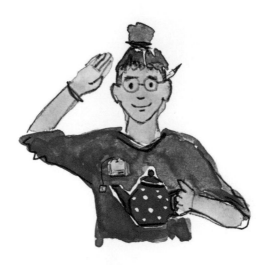

## Is your deadline movable?

Even if you've moved it already, it's always better to reach out and be open about your progress, rather than push yourself to the point of mental breakdown, only to turn in half-baked work. If there are people around you insisting the work must be done immediately, it's okay to question why.

## Ask for help.

You are probably not asking for help because you are embarrassed. Maybe you promised you'd have finished this thing yesterday. Maybe you said you could do it alone. Maybe you think asking for help says 'something' about you. All of that is total crap. If you're so buried in work you can hardly breathe, the people around you will naturally want to help. So let them.

## I work alone and there's nobody to help me!

Perhaps a friend or family member can help you with a simple but necessary task, like preparing, sorting or organising. Perhaps you know an aspiring talent who would be interested in some work experience. Or maybe you could badger a fellow freelancer to work with you for moral support. Performing better when you're working alongside others is a phenomenon called 'social facilitation' and is like having a running buddy who helps you push yourself.

## Prioritise and reschedule.

If you don't have a to-do list, jot one down now. Start by considering the brief, objectives or intention, and break the exact requirements of your project into small, manageable chunks. Then order these by urgency – or separate them into 'must-haves' and 'nice-to-haves'. In other words, let yourself do only what really matters and cross off or reschedule the rest. Allot your available time to the items remaining on your list. And stick to it.

## Can you take other work off your plate?

Are you volunteering, helping someone else, working on a personal project or trying to hustle a side gig? Put off any extra work until you have the time, space and mental clarity. Send a message to the people you promised to help and explain your situation. They will understand.

## Are your standards too high?

I know it's frustrating when this happens, but when you can't seem to actualise a brilliant idea by the deadline, it's time to go to Plan B. Perhaps you thought you could write a really funny conference speech but the jokes failed to materialise. It sucks, but you're now better off doing a simple version, rather than tearing your hair out over the original idea.

## Are you letting yourself become distracted?

Be strict with yourself. Get off social media. Turn off your access to wifi or go somewhere without it. At home, I bury my phone under my pillow. There's also software available that can lock down your devices and help you focus, like Freedom, Anti-Social, Forest or FocusWriter. If you're stuck in a noisy workspace, try listening to classical music or white noise through headphones. (Related: no, those mugs do not need to be cleaned right now.)

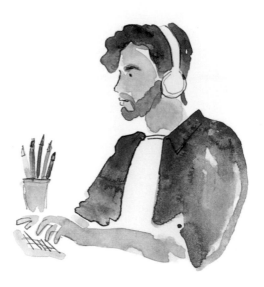

### Try the Pomodoro Technique.

Work in highly focussed bursts of 25 minutes, followed by a 5-minute break. Rinse and repeat. Set a timer on your phone or use a free app, like Focus Keeper.

### Is it really that you have run out of ideas?

Skip to page 69.

### Do your worst.

Give yourself permission to suck. Something is always better than nothing, and something often turns into quite a good thing with some refining.

## You may decide to pull an all-nighter.

This is not recommended, nor is it something to make habitual, but if you have truly exhausted all options and you feel you must work all night, be smart about it. Load up on protein-heavy snacks, lots of water and the occasional caffeinated drink. Avoid sugar highs. Take periodic breaks to stretch and move your body. Listen to focus music. And, most importantly, make tomorrow as restful as possible.

## You may have to accept it is not possible to do this work at this time.

Never sacrifice your health and wellbeing for your work. Do not buy into the myth that successful people must suffer and work insane hours to be authentic. If there is no way to finish your work right now, let yourself accept defeat so you can learn from this experience.

## Figure out how long you really need to work.

It's tempting to please people by saying yes to everything that comes your way and trying to do it as fast as possible. In reality it's better to slightly under-promise so you can always over-deliver. If you're freelance and have a client who insists on tight turnarounds, explain that you will need to charge a higher rate or rush fee. Often this is all it takes to get a reasonable deadline.

## Are you secretly addicted to panic?

Do you find yourself messing about, getting absolutely no work done, until you're suffocating under the pressure of a deadline? The thing to do here is accept you secretly love the delicious pain of a deadline – and schedule in a bunch of your own before the real one hits. If there's some part of your brain that won't accept these as real deadlines, see if you can get someone else to hold you to account. If it's not someone you work with, you could even promise them cake or wine for every deadline you crash. (One of my friends gave me a cheque for £1,000 that she'd made out to a lobbying group she despised, and told me to cash it if she didn't send me her screenplay within six weeks!)

# I'M PANICKING ABOUT A MEETING

The lead-up to an important meeting never fails to give me an identity crisis. It's clear to me that we do not live in a meritocracy and that structural bias creeps into every facet of society, so I start to panic that I will be treated unfairly because I'm a woman, because I have anxiety or because I have an accent. You might be worried about other, even worse, structural biases, like racism, ableism or trans- or homophobia. Or you might simply be worried you'll wear a stupid outfit.

The truth is, none of the advice in this section should be necessary. We are slowly overturning the system just by being here and presenting our authentic selves. However, if you're already feeling fragile and burnt out, here are some tips to help avoid a full-on pre-meeting panic.

## Pick your outfit in advance.

Stave off the dreaded Clothing Crisis by planning your outfit the night before – and sticking to it. The irritating thing with modern work is that you do not necessarily want to look like 'a suit' but you don't want to look unprofessional either. I find it is better to lean towards traditional professional attire, with creative, cultural or personal touches. Consider adding a 'conversation piece' – something interesting with a sense of humour or a bit of story to it, like bright socks, bold jewellery or something vintage.

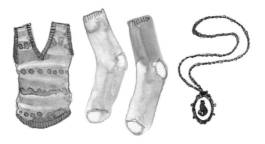

## Rehearse, but don't obsess.

Practise your self-introduction, your pitch and your small talk out loud so that it sounds natural. Don't try to memorise exact lines, just the general gist, flow and tone. Rehearsing out loud can feel weird at first, but I like to think of it as getting out all your awkward word vomit – so it doesn't end up splattered all over the poor souls in your meeting.

## Bring a notepad.

A notepad is a fantastic prop for awkward silences. When in doubt, nod sagely and jot down the last thing that was said. These notes can sometimes spark ideas for more questions to ask. Do not use or look at your phone unless specifically directed to do so.

## Arrive early.

Give yourself time to settle your thoughts in a nearby café or in the reception area. Plan your trip in advance, anticipating traffic and transport delays.

## Fake it 'til you make it.

Although the idea that you can boost your confidence by striking a 'power stance' has been widely discredited, you can still make a huge impact on the way you feel and the way you are received by using open body language, eye contact and a warm smile. Don't worry if it doesn't feel quite like 'you'. Nothing about this situation is natural. Just use it to get yourself through the door with a smile.

## Make it a conversation.

Feel free to let the other side speak first or start with small talk. If you feel put on the spot, respond with a question. Ask them to explain what they are looking for. It's okay to answer specific questions with 'I can get right back to you on that.'

## Drink water and chew gum.

Japanese researchers found that chewing gum for over ten minutes relieves stress[19]. Drinking water is just plain good for you and helps prevent headaches. (Although do nip off for a 'safety wee' before the meeting!)

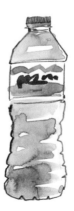

## They want you to be your best.

Have you ever been to an amateur stand-up night and felt second-hand cringe for a comic who is bombing? Whoever you're meeting with doesn't want you to bomb either. This is not a battle and they are not your enemy. They are rooting for you.

## Slow down and deepen your voice.

A common side effect of nerves is to start talking at rapid speed or in a squeaky pitch, usually because you're tensing your neck muscles and your throat's gone all clacky and dry. It's hard to tell that you are doing this, so make a mental note to periodically stop, take a sip of water, lift your chin and relax your neck.

## Involve your audience.

No, I don't mean pull them up on stage and saw them in half. (Though that would be a hell of a pitch.) Talk about 'we' and 'us'. Ask if you've missed anything, or how your idea could be made stronger. If you can bring the room from passive listening to active involvement, you've already started to win them over.

# I CAN'T SAY NO.
# I CAN'T SWITCH OFF

Most of us have a strong sense of fear around the idea of refusal – especially in the workplace. We fear we will be seen as lazy, unwilling and uncompetitive, perhaps even that we will be fired. We fear these things even as workaholism drives us to distraction, sleeplessness and diminishing returns on our productivity. And we fear that some of us can more easily afford to say no than others, because of things like wealth, age, race and sex. But when it comes to burnout, you can physically do only so much, so you *must* learn how to refuse in order to survive long term. It's not fun. It's not optional. It's a life skill.

## Double-check your gut reaction.

Are you even letting yourself consider saying no? Think about your reason for turning something down. It is probably completely acceptable. All you need to do is think of a comfortable way to phrase it. Some people will want you to obsequiously gush about how badly you wish you could have helped. Others will prefer a blunt, upfront answer.

## Consider a conditional affirmative.

If you really can't stomach the idea of a flat-out no, put some conditions on your yes. For example, that you could do it if there were more time, if you had assistance, or if there were a different approach. That way you're happy if the work goes ahead, and if it doesn't, it's the other side who said no.

## Outsource the boring bits.

Don't get worked up about things that aren't going to play a huge role in your career. Outsource as many non-work-related tasks as you can, whether through services or help from family and friends. Perhaps you could hire an accountant or cleaning services, or organise to have groceries delivered. Local libraries are a treasure trove of free services, like CV checking, business advice and supervised homework clubs for kids. Perhaps your family could pitch in more with chores, or you could devise a 'ride sharing' system with colleagues. The hardest part is asking.

## Set boundaries.

Be clear about the times of day that are appropriate for you to do work and switch off your access to devices outside those hours. If you work from home or you often need to bring work home, designate a space that is for work and work *only*. When you're in the space, you work. And when you're not, you don't. It sounds simple, but when you work anywhere and everywhere in your home, it becomes more and more difficult to relax in those places. Particularly the bed. Beds are for sleep and sex, not filing tax returns. End of story!

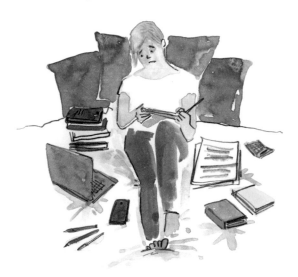

## Dial down the perfectionism.

Don't make more work for yourself by going over and over things until they're 'perfect'. (Spoiler: nothing in life is perfect, and that's what makes it so beautiful.) Learn to recognise the point at which you have overworked something.

## Don't define yourself by your productivity.

You do not have to be 'useful' to be worthy. We live in an economy that pressures us to commodify, optimise and justify every last second of our lives – even in the way we curate the image of our holidays and free time on social media. (Stanford University professor Jenny Odell calls this the 'attention economy' and she has written a fascinating book about how to resist it called *How to Do Nothing*.)

As a freelancer, one of the traps I fall into is feeling like I'm not working hard enough, simply because I can work in my pyjamas or take an afternoon stroll in exchange for working a little later. Remind yourself that you are a human soul, not a job title. You're working as hard as you need to. And you don't have to spend every waking moment hustling just to prove it.

# I'VE RUN OUT OF IDEAS

When your brain feels fried to a crisp, it's hard to think of anything – let alone a good idea. But what if your job relies on problem-solving, analysing or just generally coming up with stuff? Almost every job requires creativity, but many of us never learn how to cultivate it. Step one: stop banging your head on the desk. Good. That's one fantastic idea already! Step two: read on.

## You are creative.

It doesn't matter if you 'just' built the spreadsheet, 'just' laid out the tea or 'only' handle customer problems. Congratulations, you're being creative. Sure, most of us can't hang our work in a gallery, but that doesn't mean we should ignore our entire creative skillset. It's a unique human gift. Acknowledge it. Nurture it. Believe in it. Because ideas are fragile little things and telling yourself you're 'not creative' does nothing but kill them on the spot.

'The creative adult is the child who survived.'

_____

**URSULA K. LE GUIN**

## Are you criticising everything you do?

Ah, yes: *everything I come up with is crap, I am a fraud and everybody knows it.* When this helpful mood strikes, frame and distance your thoughts as if they were said by someone else. Use phrases like, 'I see that I am...'; for example, 'I see that I'm telling myself I am a lazy little turd.' When said out loud like this, I nearly always laugh and the power of that negative thought is destroyed.

## Are you waiting for The Perfect Idea?

Let's rip that plaster off now: it's never coming. And trust me, this is a good thing. It means that somewhere in that jumble of accidental thoughts, instincts and what-if-we-justs, you've already got something you can work into a brilliant idea. You just have to let it start out flawed.

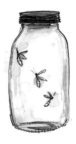

## Do you always use the same process?

There's a saying often misattributed to Albert Einstein: 'Insanity is doing the same thing over and over again and expecting a different result.' I'm afraid I have no idea who said it, but it is a useful reminder when it comes to generating ideas. Sometimes we get so set in our ways we can't see we have tried only one old method for coming up with stuff.

Where you really need ideas is in the *way* you spark them in the first place. If you tend to sit at your desk staring at a blank document, get up and move around with a notepad or rearrange notecards on a table. If you tend to bounce around the internet looking for inspiration, try visiting a library or museum. And if you work alone, why not collaborate this time?

## Are your parameters too broad or too narrow?

You may be trying to create a Big Universal Thing or a Very Very Very Particular Thing. Neither are useful approaches. If you find yourself casting about wildly, set yourself a framework. If you hate rules, don't worry, you can break them! The point is that restrictions spark ideas. If, however, you are trying to create something really specific, you are probably stifling yourself with an impossible task. Start again. Let the weirdness in. Wander through the left field. You can always rein in a wild idea.

## Try an Oblique Strategy.

Created by Brian Eno, Oblique Strategies are cards printed with thought-provoking phrases like 'emphasise the flaws', 'only one element of each kind' or 'make something implied more definite'. There's no set way to use the cards – you could pick out one or arrange a few randomly together. The idea is to see how the questions or statements affect your work. You could even write your own set of cards.

## Create a productivity playlist.

Music is a great way to get in the zone. Creating the perfect playlist for your project can be a surprisingly effective way to jog ideas and keep you focussed.

## Shake up your schedule or your surroundings.

Get out of your workspace and your mindset – physically. Schedule that meeting in a different place. Switch desks. Walk somewhere while listening to music. Stretch. Meditate. Even something as simple as sitting on the floor can be enough to change your perspective.

## When did you last 'fill the tank'?

This is my phrase for the raw material that swills around in your brain and eventually bumps together, forming ideas. (Neil Gaiman calls it composting.) The important thing is, you shouldn't keep draining the same well for your material. Read something you'd usually avoid. Watch different kinds of movies. Talk to new people. Listen to strange music. Use someone else's process. Get up and *go* somewhere.

## Are you dealing with personal problems?

Psychotherapist Dennis Palumbo says creative block is really 'a self-protective mechanism, one probably "installed" in child-hood, that's continuing in your adult life'[20]. He says block is best conceptualised as a signpost, pointing out the issues, feelings or habits you need to resolve to move forward.

# I CAN'T HANDLE SETBACKS

So you didn't get on the scheme. That pitch didn't work out. You were passed over for a promotion. If there's anything more guaranteed to whack up the heat on your burnout, it's getting a big fat no. But it's not all bad. You might not be able to see it immediately, but setbacks are usually more like signposts. You just have to figure out which way they're pointing you.

## Take some time to be upset.

It's okay if a rejection makes you feel sad, worthless, frustrated or even angry – as long as you acknowledge that these are just raw feelings that will pass. Find a healthy way to let the rage out so the relief can rush in.

## Rest and recharge.

It can be tempting to get right back up on the horse, but that's exactly how you double down on your burnout. Time is your friend. It's not too late and you are not too old.

## It's rarely personal.

Unless you've done something completely unprofessional, you won't get rejected just because someone doesn't like you. It usually means your work wasn't the right fit, wasn't up to the right standard or did not fulfil the requirements. Try not to extrapolate from any rejection that you are a failure. Instead, put your work or application away for at least a month, then come back to it with fresh eyes and see if you can learn anything about how it could have been better.

If, however, you feel you have been discriminated against, consider complaining directly to the top of the company or bringing in a mediator to discuss your concerns. You can call the government's Equality Advisory Support Services for information and advice.

## Collect rejections.

Change the way you think about rejections by aiming to collect a certain number of them. Applying for a new job is a great opportunity to bank at least 20. As a writer, I aim for 100 rejections a year. In his book *On Writing*, Stephen King describes hanging rejection slips on a nail on his wall until it could no longer support the weight of them all. And after that? 'I replaced the nail with a spike,' he says, 'and went on writing.'

## There's an opportunity in there somewhere.

Every great success story is paved with failures. Imagine how boring your memoir would be if you got everything right first time. Nobody wants to hear that! Every setback is an opportunity to strengthen your resolve and critically re-evaluate your work. Then look up from your feet and create a new plan for moving forward. Now take the first step.

# Famous Failures &
# Late Bloomers

**Bill Gates** was 17 when he debuted new traffic-data technology to Seattle County officials... which completely failed to work.

**Ariana Huffington** was pretty much unknown before founding the Huffington Post at age 55.

**Colonel Sanders** had his famous chicken recipe rejected over 1,000 times, before he finally founded his own franchise at age 65.

**Oprah Winfrey** was fired from her first television presenting role for being 'too emotional'.

**Soichiro Honda** had his first factory bombed by B-52s, and the second levelled in an earthquake. He sold the remains to his rival Toyota and created the Honda motorcycle.

**Alan Rickman** changed careers in his 30s and was 41 when he got his first big role in *Die Hard*.

**George Orwell** was 42 when his book *Animal Farm* finally launched his career, two decades after he began writing.

**Henry Ford** went bankrupt after his first two attempts to start a business. He was 45 when he finally created the Ford Model T.

**Vera Wang** tried figure skating and then journalism, before realising her passion was fashion at age 40.

# I FEEL PATRONISED

There's nothing more delightful than battling your way through a long day at work, only to have That Person come along and remind you that you're still rubbish. They think they're being clever, but they're like baboons shaking their inflamed red arses around the workplace, trying to let everyone know that they're the ones in control. Well, frankly, nobody has to work with a baboon arse.

## This is their issue, not yours.

At its heart, patronising is a subtle form of bullying. It's important to remind yourself that this has nothing to do with you and everything to do with the way this person sees the world. So don't give their opinion any space in your mind. You don't need criticism from someone you would never go to for advice.

## Politely put yourself back on their level.

The unfortunate truth is many people don't realise when they are patronising. Some are genuinely trying to be helpful. Others are excited about teaching and sharing. And some just need to learn how to read the room. That's why a great way to disarm a patroniser is to completely agree with them with an example of your own. This turns their 'advice' into a conversation set on equal footing. 'You're absolutely right,' you say. 'In fact, I did the same thing last year on a previous project.'

Another strategy is to slyly ask why they're telling you something, but again, framing it so you're both equally involved. 'Hey, just so I'm clear – I know how to use this software, so was there something in particular we're missing here? Let's solve that.'

## Dealing with a power play.

Some people will deliberately try to put you down to make themselves feel superior. Sometimes they'll even do it in front of others. While it's tempting to say, 'Could you please just let me speak!?' this can come off as passive-aggressive and fill the room with tension. The best route is to calmly and persistently ask your patroniser for clarification. Ask them to explain their reasoning or come up with a better alternative. Essentially, this strategy is a way of showing you're aware of their subtext. A patroniser will usually tie themselves up in knots trying not to reveal the insult they had hidden as 'helpful advice'. This strategy is also a fabulous riposte to sexist or racist jokes. Just pretend not to get it and ask them to explain why it's funny.

## This person may feel threatened by you.

In some cases, a patroniser wants to put you in your place because they're afraid of losing theirs. Sometimes it's useful to start by simply getting to know this person better and understanding where they are coming from.

## Use your body language as armour.

Have you ever tried so hard to hold your tongue that you end up saying it with your face? Don't let non-verbal cues give others an excuse to treat you badly. Ask a trusted friend to help you evaluate your communication style, tone, posture, body language and facial expressions. Perhaps you present yourself as younger, less smart or less serious than you really are.

The solution isn't changing everything about yourself. It's learning how to control the non-verbal messages you send in crucial moments. I have a tendency to use dorky slang, slump my shoulders, chew my lip and make overeager hand gestures, which can all combine to look a bit teenaged. Other common problems are poor eye contact, hands kept in pockets, obsessive phone checking, crossed arms, giggling, speaking in a higher pitch... not finishing sentences...

## Boss up your look.

I know this sounds a bit Hollywood Makeover Movie, but your hairstyle and clothes say as much about you as your body language. There's a cliché that is helpful here: dress for the job you want, not the job you have. Which kind of sounds like it's telling you to rock up dressed like a part-time astronaut cake-taster. But the truth is, it never hurts to dress like you mean business. Even if you wear a uniform to work, wear it as best you can.

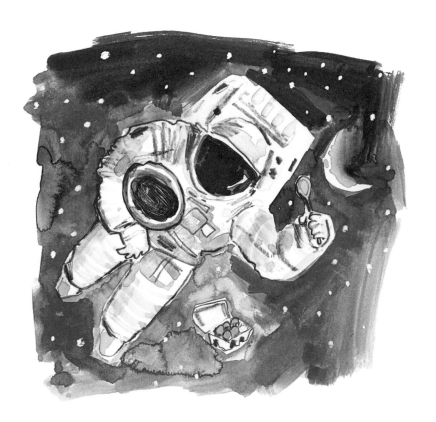

## Promote yourself from Tea Bitch.

If you're always the first person asked to fire up the kettle, take the minutes or organise the birthday cakes, make a firm but light-hearted comment that reminds everyone they should be pulling their weight. Something like, 'I'll get this one, but you're doing the next one!' If it's your boss who keeps asking, and you feel there are others on your level who should be helping, use your freshly ordained organisational authority to create a roster. Nobody can fight with a roster. That's the real tea.

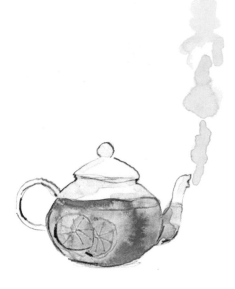

# I PROCRASTINATE. I HAVE NO MOTIVATION

Procrastination and poor motivation are tell-tale signs of burnout. They can happen separately, or they can team up together to volley negative thoughts right into your brain like the world's most evil tennis doubles. Either way, this fun scenario boils down to the same two questions. Why should I even do this? And why now?

## You need a reason to do the work.

And it needs to be more than get paid. If you're struggling to get anything done, it's probably because you feel no personal connection to the work, so it feels like a chore. Now, the work may well be a chore, but if you can give yourself a reason and context, it will at least feel worth doing.

In the army, they call this 'unifying purpose'. And frankly, if the army can find an answer to 'WAR! WHAT IS IT GOOD FOR?' which gets countless talented individuals to risk their lives in all sorts of scary ways, then you can find a reason to do your chore.

If you asked Simone Biles why she's doing all those repetitive gymnastics drills, she's not going to say, 'To get through the day.' She's going to say, 'To win gold at the Olympics.' So what's your Olympics? What's your war? What's your dream? It doesn't have to be big, it just has to be real.

## What if I don't have a dream job?

Your big dream doesn't have be a career. In fact, it is probably healthier if it isn't. Deciding the kind of person you want to be, the kind of relationships you want to cultivate or the kind of experiences you want to have in life is just as much The Dream as anything else.

## Set specific goals.

Say you want to be a famous cinematographer. That's a great dream, but it says nothing about how to get there. Unromantic though it may seem, the pathway to your dream is a series of small, specific, measurable goals. A great way to figure out your goals is to use the phrase 'in order to' until it builds a logical sentence. Even if some of your goals are purely mercenary – 'pull pints in order to earn enough money in order to shoot my first short film' – if you're clear why you're working for each goal, motivation comes naturally.

## Break your day into manageable steps.

Once you know why you're showing up at work, now you need to figure out how to get through it. Make a step-by-step list of what it will take to finish the day's work. This not only gives you the smug satisfaction of crossing it all off as you go, but also helps build momentum. I like to draw little circles next to the items on my list, filling in half the circle when I've started a step, and the whole thing when it's done.

## Reward the little wins.

One of the problems with small steps and little goals is that nobody else cares about them, so they can start to feel thankless and worthless. When you do set a goal, set a reward to go with it – making sure to recognise the sort of reward system that actually works for you.

If you like things to feel official, think of it like designing your own personal Advent calendar. Every time you achieve a certain amount, you get to open a window – and you can put whatever you like behind that window. Even if all you can think about is binge-watching the latest series of *Queer Eye*, put that behind your window today.

The important thing is to *celebrate* every accomplishment with kindness, creating positive associations with your work – not punish yourself for the times you slip up, which will be many and often. (Because you're normal.)

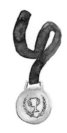

### Do some smart procrastination.

Sometimes achieving a small semi-related task can give you the motivation to get stuck in for real. Maybe you could read things related to your task, organise your files or get all of those emails out of the way.

### If the carrot isn't working, try the stick.

Imagine somebody making headlines for exactly what you want to do. Now beat them to it.

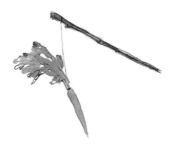

### Try a career or life coach.

It can seem strange paying someone to tell you what to do, but it means you can really focus on what you do best without worrying if it's right. If this is cost prohibitive, ask a friend, relative or colleague if they're willing to sit down with you and help give you this perspective.

## All work (even creative work) is a routine habit.

It's easy to procrastinate or give yourself excuses if you're trying to do something difficult or creative. But ultimately, work is work, and we can't be waiting around for some mythical muse. We need to be able to get stuck in all day, every day, even when we don't feel so great.

Learn how to show up. If you don't have working hours, set your own – say nine to five – and make sure you're in your space, ready to go, nine on the dot. Part of developing healthy habits is training yourself to show up and keep at it for eight hours a day.

## Those negative voices are not always your own.

You may be hearing an overly critical parent, toxic friend or unhelpful boss. A great way to get these out of your head is to imagine a funny creature who says them to you. I invented a horse named Hot Pants – one of those fancy, prance-y, dance-y ones with the bizarre dumpling-bun hairstyles. My negative voices are sometimes still there, but they're a hell of a lot easier to deal with coming from such a silly horse.

## Learn how to 'run five miles to the door'.

For the brilliant TV showrunner Shonda Rhimes, getting to that good place, where you're feeling all inspired and motivated and loving it, first requires 'running five miles just to get to the door'[21]. In other words, you can't simply sit down and expect ideas to happen. You need to warm up to the task, get that energy flowing, and jog five miles before you can really start to race.

For Shonda, learning to run five miles requires two things. First, a comfortable, ergonomic, (ideally) distraction-free space. And second, a simple way to hop on the starting blocks. This is a small activity you never seem to mind doing that helps you ease into the work. For me, it's reading over the work I wrote the day before. I tell myself, 'Don't worry if you have no ideas, all you have to do right now is read.' And somehow, I can begin.

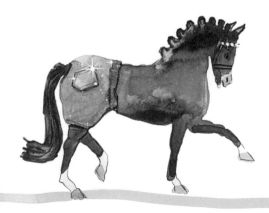

# Emergency Chocolate

As a kid I was fascinated by the stories of Japanese samurai who would make sure they always carried an umeboshi (sour pickled plum) on their adventures. It was said that umeboshi could combat battle fatigue and that the mere thought of it would help your mouth water if you were thirsty.

Umeboshi aren't so easy to come by in London, so I always pack emergency chocolate rations. When I find myself beginning to stress or worry, the mere thought of a chocolate treat is often enough to give me the confidence to carry on that little bit further. I've scoffed chocolate on planes, trains, before meetings, walking down the street, in the back of taxis... I've even been known to escape to the loo just to smash a whole bar because I've turned up to a social event that I thought would involve food but everyone keeps ordering drinks. It's a truly indispensable item.

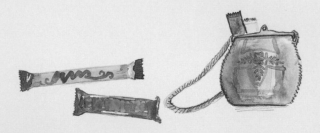

# I CAN'T STAND WORKING WITH THAT PERSON

Where would office sitcoms be without all the plonkers, knobs and wet blankets who lurk in our workplaces? In the real world, working with these people is no laughing matter – especially when you're already frazzled and exhausted. First things first: it is perfectly okay not to be friends with everyone. Finding a way to work with someone is not the same as actually liking them.

## Don't take it personally.

Unless you're being bullied (see page 98), a difficult person isn't going out of their way just to annoy you. Their behaviour will usually stem from a strain in their life, such as anger, frustration, insecurity or depression. It may not be okay for them to act the way they do, but it's healthy to acknowledge it's not just because of you.

### Try to learn a few things about them.

The more time we spend with people, the more we tend to like them[22]. If you need to, be cynical about it and imagine yourself as a spy extracting secret knowledge to help you better understand what makes this person tick.

### Acknowledge the good stuff.

It sounds a bit like dealing with a toddler, but it works. Acknowledging good behaviours and changes while ignoring the bad can create a positive feedback loop that improves your relationship.

### Do you really hate them or your own situation?

When you're stressed beyond belief, dread going to work, or something is going badly in your personal life, sometimes even the nicest people come across as monsters. That guy organising a pub lunch must be a sleaze. That girl offering cupcakes is trying to fatten you up. That manager with the suspiciously neutral expression definitely has it in for you. If you find yourself struggling to get along with lots of people, you need to check yourself out first. Or as the saying goes, 'When everything around you smells like poo, check under your own shoe.'

# How to Handle Those People

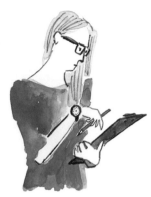

## Mindy the Micromanager

There's only one way to do things and that's Mindy's way. This sort of person is often insecure and stressed about delivering, so the trick is not to push back, but to offset the worrying. If you rebel against it, Mindy could decide you can't be trusted and only get more involved. So build trust by figuring out what she cares about and delivering in those areas. A little flattery helps: 'I see how much pressure you're under. How can I help?' It's also useful to over-report your progress.

Another trick is to sit down with her at the beginning of the project and agree on how she will track it, gently pushing back on her micromanaging tendencies by reminding her you'll handle the minutiae, so she can focus on the big strategy.

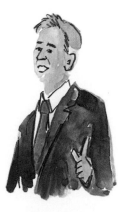

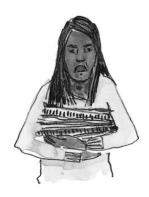

## Brian the Blagger

Fantastic at repeating whatever was just said and an absolute ninja with delegating, Brian knows how to talk the talk without walking the walk. The hardest part about dealing with a Brian is that everyone else thinks he's doing a great job, while you pick up his slack. The trick is to re-delegate. Explain that after some careful thinking, you've all realised *he's* the one best placed to do the work.

## Ingrid the Impatient

Ingrid expects you to instantly understand everything, even if nothing was ever explained or you were literally hired yesterday. This person is usually bad at managing their own time, which makes them worry they will now have to spend all of their time helping you. Show empathy for their busy schedule and explain you will be able to do everything they need if they just point you to the right information and resources.

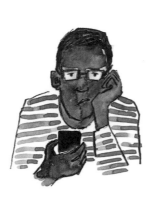

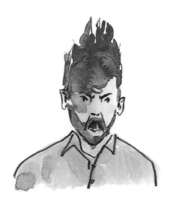

## Derek the Dead Weight

How is Derek still employed? It is an unsolved mystery that has now become your problem, because you need Derek to actually do something. With Derek, it's best to be clear and direct with your request, or refer it to his manager.
If you *are* his manager, this is about creating reasons for him to care about the work and implementing more transparency so that everyone can see who actually does what.

## Hector the Hothead

Hector's problem is that he brings all his other problems to work. Emotional people aren't thinking straight, so try to identify what is upsetting him using neutral phrases like, 'Hold on a second, what's this about?' If Hector gets aggressive, psychiatrist Dr Mark Goulston advises to let him finish his outburst, wait pointedly for two to four seconds, and say, 'Could you run that by me again?'[23] This shows the room you are on to Hector and forces him to hear what he's saying.

# When it's bullying, harassment or discrimination

If a colleague has gone beyond annoying and is behaving in a way that makes you feel uncomfortable or unfairly treated, you should consider pursuing more serious recourse. You're automatically protected against harassment and discrimination thanks to the Equality Act 2010, and when it comes to bullying, consult your company's policy. (If they don't have one, use the default procedure at ACAS, a public body that works with employers and employees to improve workplace relationships.) Discuss this with your HR department to decide how you would like the issue handled, or contact ACAS for free advice:

**ACAS**
Weekdays 8am to 6pm
acas.org.uk
0300 123 1100
18001 0300 123 1100 (for texts)

# EVERYTHING HURTS. I'M IN TERRIBLE SHAPE

Whether you're sat hunched in front of a screen or standing on aching feet, any stationary posture is bad for your health[24]. Working from home can be just as painful, with 51% of people experiencing injuries or aches and pains as a result of their working environment[25]. Here's how to bring a spot of comfort to your workplace.

### Let there be daylight.

Natural light is good for you. Working near a window gives you an average of 46 minutes more sleep each night[26].

### Get up and move it, move it.

The British Chiropractic Association recommends taking a break to move around every 20–30 minutes[27]. Get up to make a tea, or walk around every time you make a phone call. Take your lunch break outside if you can, incorporating a walk.

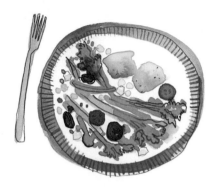

### Eat healthily but don't diet.

You know the drill! Lots of vegetables, fruit and protein, and a lot less of those refined carbs and sugars. I'm no dietitian, but if you don't have specific allergies or requirements, I find healthy eating works best with an 'all-in-moderation' rule. That is, eat absolutely anything you want, but only an appropriate amount. Also, choose colourful veggies and fruits. If you struggle to keep up with cooking, try jumping on the meal-prep trend and batch cook your meals.

### Book a masseur or physiotherapist.

For stubborn aches and pains, try a Thai hot herbal compress massage, or physiotherapy.

## Protect your circadian rhythm.

If you want to get real about your health, stop beginning and ending the day staring at your phone. Excessive screen use can cause vision fatigue, dry eyes and headaches. And if you use a device right before bed, the blue light exposure reduces your production of melatonin, which creates difficulty sleeping[28]. Changes in sleep patterns then mess up your 'body clock' – your circadian rhythm – which can have devastating repercussions because your body clock controls both your wakefulness and the individual functions of your organs[29]. So if you're feeling sluggish and not sleeping too well, put yourself on a strict device detox.

## Minimise eye damage and fatigue.

All digital devices emit blue wavelength light, which reaches deeper into the eye than UV light and, with continued exposure over time, causes retinal damage[30]. There are four ways to help protect your eyes and I suggest doing all of them. The first is to install a melanopic light app, such as f.lux (justgetflux.com), which makes the light of your screen match the room you're in. The next is to apply light-filtering screen stickers to all of your devices. Third, ensure the ambient light in your workspace is only about half of what you'd expect in an office. And finally, commit to wearing computer glasses or 'anti-reflective' glasses while you use any device.

## Incorporate easy ways to exercise.

The trick here is to pick something you like doing anyway. It could be walking your dog, bowling or trying to learn how to dance like a robot. These days there's a class or YouTube video for just about anything. I know it can be hard to find the enthusiasm if you never had that kind of upbringing, but it's not really good enough just to say, 'I'm not sporty.' You want to be able to walk when you're retired, right? That fitness starts now.

Signing up for a set of classes is a great way to force your motivation, too. Not only have you already paid for them, but you'll find yourself building a new social circle full of people who love your activity as much as you do.

## Practise stretching and spinal care.

Sometimes I get so stuck into my work that I hunch over my desk despite the fact that it's all set up to be ergonomic. That's why it's important to wind down the day with stretches or yoga. I highly recommend Kit Laughlin's Daily Five stretches and Yoga with Adriene, both available for free online. For a more intense release, I lie on a lacrosse ball for 'trigger point' massage in my hips and glutes, or use a foam roller on my back and quads. It all sounds a bit brutal, but with practice and some deep breathing, you'll learn that 'hurts so good!' feeling of muscle release.

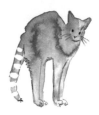
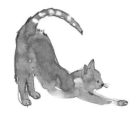

# Kit Laughlin's Daily Five

### The first stretch is to relax

The crucial thing about stretching, says Kit Laughlin, is that it starts with relaxation. Don't just hit the floor and crank yourself into these poses — you'll do more harm than good. 'Cats do not experience burnout,' he says. 'We humans have unconsciously learned to be tense, so conscious effort must be made to relax and discharge that tension.' To get ready to stretch, you could use the breathing exercises on page 35, or try one of Kit's audio relaxation and meditation classes, available for free at: stretchtherapy.net/audios

### Hold each stretch for ten relaxed breaths.

## Spinal Flexion (cat pose variation)

Sit down and hook your hands or arms under your knees, then roll back so you are balanced on your pelvis. Now slump your back and drop your head forward, creating a stretch along your upper and middle back.

## Spinal Extension (baby cobra)

Lie on your front and place your forearms by your sides. Push up your upper body, keeping your forearms and hands flat on the floor, creating an upper back arch. Be sure to consciously relax your lower back and push up from your arm muscles — never pull up from your back muscles.

## Spinal Rotation (supine twist)

Lie on your back with your legs straight, then bend one of your knees, keeping the foot on the ground. Let this knee fall over the other leg and on to the ground, while reaching your arms out to both sides. Repeat on the opposite side.

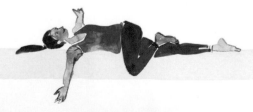

### Lateral Flexion (gate pose variation)

Kneel with your knees hip-width apart and raise one arm in the air, reaching over into a side stretch. Repeat on the opposite side.

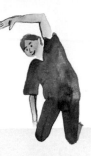

### Seated Piriformis (fire log pose variation)

Sit cross-legged on the floor. Notice which knee is on top and use the opposite elbow to hook around it and pull the knee towards you, letting your pelvis roll forward as you lift your chest along your leg, stretching the piriformis. Repeat on the opposite side.

### Optional Hip Flexor Stretch (lizard pose variation)

Kneel on one knee with the other leg bent in front at a 90° angle. Lean forward, putting your hands on the floor for support, and inch your front foot forward so that it is in front of both your hands and your knee. Now inch your other knee backward as far as you can. To create the stretch, straighten your back and pull yourself forward. Repeat on the opposite side.

### Optional Neck Sequence

Kit's colleague Liv has recorded a sequence of neck stretches that are perfect for 'desk jockeys' because you can do them any time, sitting in your seat: youtu.be/bQG13mB23CU

## Designate an ergonomic work environment.

Your employer should really be providing this for you. But if you're freelance or your 'workspace' is just a rotation of sofas, beds and wooden coffee-shop seats, it's time to give your body some TLC. You need to create a quality 'work only' space that flips your brain into 'work mode' *and* helps you stay healthy while you do it. Find yourself an adjustable ergonomic chair – or failing that, orthopaedic cushions. If you use a computer, make sure your screen is at eye level and your keyboard is at elbow level, as shown in the diagram below.

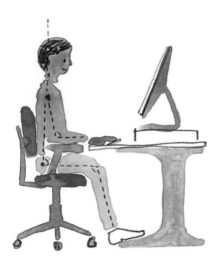

# The Burnout-free Workplace

79% of employees suffer from mild, moderate or severe burnout[31]. It can seem like a personal thing, but it wouldn't happen if we had healthy workplaces and cultures. Things like deep breathing, wellness walks and gratitude are wonderful, but these strategies alone cannot (and should not) be expected to battle the demon that is burnout. What's more, bad workplace design kills productivity by 20% and turnover by up to 15%[32]. So what should we do?  This section uses the latest data to help employers implement The Burnout-free Workplace.

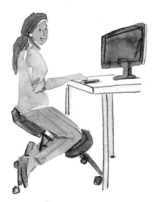

## Workstations

Designate one ergonomic workstation per employee. So-called 'hotdesking' may save you money, but it increases distrust, distractions, uncooperative behaviour and negative relationships[33].

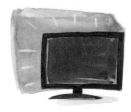

## Screens

Protect eyesight with melanopic light apps and screen stickers. Encourage screen breaks and non-screen-based working.

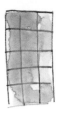
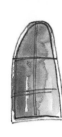

### Lighting

Put workstations near windows and provide customisable lighting.

### Air Quality

Manage $CO_2$ levels with proper ventilation for a 101% boost in cognition[34].

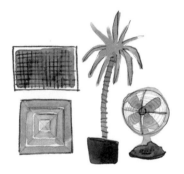

### Noise

Stripped-back warehouses may look cool, but noise creates a 66% drop in performance[35]. Minimise distractions with sound-absorbing materials and quiet zones.

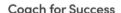

### Coach for Success

Acknowledge contributions and provide progression. Four in five employees who leave their jobs cite lack of appreciation as one of the reasons[36].

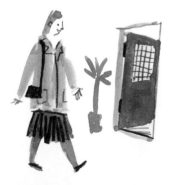

### Proper Breaks

No more lunches al-desko. Something as little as a five-minute walk boosts mood and counters fatigue[37].

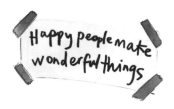

Happy people make wonderful things

### Identity and Purpose

Include everyone in defining the ideal place to work, supported by a unifying purpose.

### The Golden Rule

Treat others how you would like to be treated.

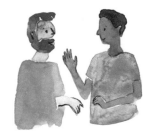

### Clear and Fair

Be clear in what you expect and fair in how you enforce it.

### Listen and Learn

Create channels for everyone to be heard, with a process of continual refinement. Companies where employees feel connected to management produce three times as much revenue growth.*

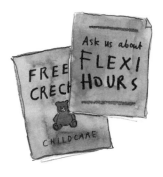

Ask us about FLEXI HOURS

FREE CRECH

CHILDCARE

### Perks, Not Piffle

Beanbags and ping-pong tables are cute, but companies that invest in their employees instead of gimmicks tend to outperform their competitors[38].

* A fantastic place to get started on building a better workplace culture is the organisation Great Place to Work: greatplacetowork.com

# LONG-TERM PROBLEMS

'Failure is unimportant. It takes courage to make a fool of yourself.'

CHARLIE CHAPLIN

# WHAT IF I'M NOT GOOD ENOUGH? I FEEL LIKE I WILL NEVER 'MAKE IT'

First of all, what does this question even mean? Nobody is ever provably 'good enough' because there is no giant test that tells you if you passed or failed at life. There's just a long road of challenges, obstacles and opportunities, all of which will determine your unique career journey.

You may have set yourself specific goals to achieve, and that's great. But if it takes you two hundred shots to get a goal, it doesn't mean you're not 'good enough'. It means you've grown two hundred times and you ain't no damn quitter! Don't mistake feelings of burnout for failure.

## Who are you comparing yourself to?

Do you idolise a certain person in your industry who perhaps achieved everything you want at the ripe old age of 25? It's important to be inspired by the work of others, but it will never make sense to try to map their career trajectory on to your own. They made the right choices for them at the time, but you are a completely different person with completely different skills and output. Focus on the opportunities you can find or build right now, or you will risk waiting your entire life for a 'big break' that never comes.

## Check your imposter syndrome.

This is a surprisingly common phenomenon where, despite all the evidence to the contrary, you believe deep down that you are a fraud and that one day you're going to be 'found out'. Some people call this the 'fraud police'. It's an ingrained mental cycle that is typically linked to things like family expectations, self-esteem, perfectionism, racial identity and breaking into new environments. Recognise that you're only playing mind games with yourself and that you need to open your eyes to the success you've had, while you reconnect with your motivations for going forward. If you can't quite do it for yourself right now, imagine holding the door open for others like you.

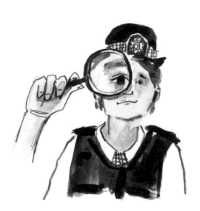

## Why do you do what you do?

The honest truth is it's extremely rare to get to the top of any career. So you need to be sure that you love what you do. Fame and fortune might be the icing, but love and passion should be your cake.

## Where were you six months ago?

You will have improved, trust me. Even if you are in a mood where you're refusing to acknowledge it, you'll have worked on new things that will have naturally developed your skills. And even if you have literally taken six months off work, you will have filled your energy tank, improved your state of mind and put yourself in the position to strike back stronger than ever.

## Release that pressure valve.

Okay, I confess. I hate this advice. I'm always deciding I 'must' achieve certain things by certain dates or I should give up. It's an attempt at motivating myself, but all it does is add so much pressure I can barely think, and then triggers a tsunami of disappointment when inevitably I fail. So take it from me: you don't have to be prolific or famous or young to be successful. You just have to be you.

'The sweet potato does not need to say how sweet it is.'

MAORI PROVERB

# I HATE NETWORKING

Yep. Me too. Networking is a pyroclastic hell realm that privileges the showman over the craftsman. But while we wait for society to develop a new alternative for introverts, the truth is, modern work (and especially freelancing) puts you in a position where you will regularly need to meet people to work with and work for. So here's how to get through an event alone.

## Plan some 'safe activities'.

Get yourself through the door with a game plan that helps you look and feel at ease being alone. I say things to myself like, 'First I'm going to get my badge, then I'm going to buy a tea, then I'm going read through the whole flyer.' Every event is different, but if, before you even walk in the door, you can think of three things to do when you're in the room, you'll never have to go through that excruciating loitering phase.

## Find someone else in your situation.

You can do it. Ask a similarly alone person a simple question, such as 'Have you been here before?' or 'Do you know where we go for the... ?' If all else fails, I have genuinely had a lot of success flashing a big smile and saying something like, 'Sorry, I don't know anyone here. I'm Imogen!' People will respond to your authenticity.

## Memorise fall-back conversation starters.

Here's a few that I like to use: 'What do you do?' 'What do you love about it?' 'What brought you here today?' 'So how do you know [the host]?' 'Do you know most of the people here?' 'Horrible weather, isn't it?' 'I like your outfit.' 'What did you think about the speaker?' 'How's your day going?' 'Are you based in [Manchester]?' 'Did you come here from work?' 'Have you seen the new [Netflix series]?'

## Ask people about themselves.

If, like me, you tend to feel guarded, self-conscious and embarrassed, don't panic. Most people want to talk about themselves. Use this to your advantage. Just keep asking about their life and their opinions.

## Learn to take a compliment.

Compliments are usually an attempt at opening a conversation, but most of us will be all British about it and accidentally shut it down. If someone wants to praise something about you – even if it's superficial, like the pin on your backpack – just smile, say thanks, and think about how you could use the compliment to get to know this person.

## Don't try to show off.

Networking isn't about finding the most senior person in the room and trying to convince them to hire you on the spot. Despite the urban legends about famous people scoring their first gig from an elevator pitch, in real life I've only ever seen this approach bomb. So let yourself take all that pressure off. Networking is not about impressing people, it's about making friends. If you find yourself chatting to someone you plain don't like, just move on.

The biggest successes I've had with networking are the genuine friends I've made along the way who have put me forward for work when an opportunity arose. These are not senior people, just people who understand me.

## Take a break.

If for any reason it all gets too much, nip off to the bathroom or some similarly secluded space and let yourself have a little breather. It's okay if repeated, forced social interactions make you feel dead inside. They're terrible! Try to keep your spirits up. You're doing better than you think just by being yourself.

# I CAN'T AFFORD MY LIFE

Is there a more miserable phrase than 'financial hygiene'? At least showering has bubbles, loofahs and fruity scents. Managing your finances is just a depressing reminder that you don't earn enough, your bills are criminal, and you probably shouldn't have tried to cheer yourself up by ordering that Lego model of the International Space Station. Money management and mental health can be a vicious cycle. Worrying about affording things can worsen your mental health, which makes it harder to manage your money in the first place. So here are some simple tips for bringing the bubbles and loofahs to your finances.

# IMPROVING CASH FLOW WHEN YOU WORK ALONE

Poor cash flow is easily the worst part of working for yourself. It's also the bit I wish were more openly discussed. I often feel like my success and my security is tied to my bank balance, so when it gets low, I feel worse than embarrassed... I feel like a failure. It's important to remember that we are not a number, and that we deserve fair compensation for our work. Here are my tried-and-tested tips for combating things like late payments, undervalued work and the madly spiralling costs of modern living.

## Get an accountant.

'So, what, the first tip is spend my money on someone else?!' Well, erm, yes. It's entirely possible to do your accounts by yourself, especially in the early days, but once you're swimming in invoices and expenses and you have to pull together a year end for Queen Lizzie herself, things can get hairy. (More like rear end, am I right? Sorry, Lizzie.) The money you spend hiring an accountant not only relieves most of this headache, it gives you someone who knows how to put your business in the best financial position. If you can't afford a dedicated accountant, there are some great specialist services out there, such as Crunch Accounting.

## Protect yourself from late payments.

Before engaging a new client, ask around about their trustworthiness and responsibility. Insist new clients sign your Terms & Conditions, committing them to paying you within specific timeframes. Copywriter Caroline Gibson has a fantastic example here: www.carolinegibson.co.uk/terms-conditions

You're also legally entitled to include late fees under the total on your invoice. (You can agree on a payment date with your client, but even if you don't, the law defines 'late' as 30 days after you issued the invoice or delivered the work – whichever happened later.) Late fees are comprised of a flat fee and an interest fee. The flat rate is £40 for invoices under £1,000; £70 for invoices under £10,000; and £100 for invoices over £10,000. The additional interest fee is 8.5%, which is statutory interest (8%) plus the Bank of England base rate for business-to-business transactions (0.5%). If you're not so hot on your maths, there's a handy late payment interest calculator at payontime.co.uk

For larger clients, request a Purchase Order (PO) before beginning work, as this forms a contract between you and the client.

## Crack the whip on deadbeat clients.

If more than 30 days have passed since your payment deadline, send a polite reminder email. If that fails, follow up with a friendly phone call and a second reminder email. If this client has an accounting department, it is definitely worth calling them directly. Better yet, make friends with this person. Kindness is your weapon!

If these attempts are still ignored, try a polite but firm 'final notice' email or letter, spiced up with some legal terms. For example, stating that your work was done *quantum meruit* means you're legally entitled to be paid for what you believe to be the reasonable value of your services.

If you're still being ignored, you can pursue legal recourse but be prepared to kill the relationship. The Government's Money Claim Online service is designed for exactly this situation, and helps you save money on solicitors and debt collection agency fees: gov.uk/make-money-claim

Finally, even if a long time has gone by, try getting in touch again anyway. I once managed to get paid 18 months after a deadline just by calling up again on a whim. The accounts department were so embarrassed I was paid the next day, no questions.

In 2019, almost two-fifths of small–medium business invoices were paid late. Collectively, these businesses were owed £34 billion in late payments[39].

## Charge more and don't do free work.

Self-employed and remote working is often undervalued because it's 'fun' and 'cool'. But you're working your arse off. Charge for it! Yes, this is a confidence game. But the longer you work, the more you can charge, and the more you can charge, the more you are valued. If you feel a conversation beginning to imply you should work for free, ask, 'So what's the budget on this?' This introduces the (fair!) assumption that you'll be paid, and if they are forced to apologise that you won't be, it's easier to decline the offer.

## Get an agent or manager.

Yeah! Just go get one! Okay, I know this is a huge step, involving networking, pitching and maybe a little begging, but impressing someone so much that they legally commit to fighting your corner will be a huge boost to your confidence, worth and credibility. Plus, once you have an agent, you can have them manage your financial conversations.

## Take on more clients.

It may be that you are charging what you are worth and still not making ends meet. It's time to get back out there and rustle up more work. Ask around your network. Send a friendly email to old clients to see if they need any help. Check for job callouts online. Take a hard look at any of your own unfinished projects and whether you could get them happening again. Consider the stability of a part-time job while you build up your client list.

## Apply for grants, bursaries, schemes.

The world craves fresh new ideas, so there will be a grant, scheme or scholarship out there for you, no matter what you're into. (Okay, maybe not murderers. Nobody wants fresh new murderers.)

If you're still feeling tentative, I understand. Applications are time-consuming, confidence-draining and always feel like they 'aren't for you'. Plus, there's the looming risk of rejection. But failure isn't the opposite of success, it's part of success. When you get picked, you get a step up, and when you don't, you have a chance to learn about yourself and refine your work. Win-win.

If you're older or already experienced, don't fall into the trap of considering these opportunities beneath you. There's nothing wrong with accepting a little boost at any point in your career.

## Do a financial 'health check'.

Take a day off just to fully evaluate your earnings, bills, debts, savings and missed opportunities. Yes, this will suck. But Martin at MoneySavingExpert claims it will save you £1,000 on average, and says it's likely to be 'the best-paid day of your year': moneysavingexpert.com/family/money-help

## Be smart with what you do have.

It's not fun or sexy, but the best place to put your money is your pension, property and/or savings account. Savings are probably the easiest place to start because you can usually just call up your bank to get an account opened for these purposes. Pensions and mortgages are harder because you tend to need advisers and brokers, but if you're aiming to run a business for some time it's important to plan out how to support yourself, your family and your retirement.

## Take the doughnuts!

This Amanda Palmer phrase is a way to say that accepting help doesn't make you less authentic[40]. When Henry David Thoreau decided to remove himself from society and write in a tiny cabin in the woods, he cemented the 'starving artist' trope and inspired the novel *Into The Wild*. But there's a lot more to his story. Thoreau's cabin was built on land owned by his friend Ralph Waldo Emerson, who regularly had him over for dinner. And every Sunday, Emerson's mother and sister brought Thoreau a freshly baked basket of pastries – including his favourite doughnuts.

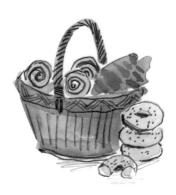

## NEGOTIATING A PAY RISE OR BENEFITS

When you just want to have a little whinge about your job, one of the most annoying responses has got to be: 'Hey, at least you're getting paid for it!' Because half the time? We're not actually getting paid what we're worth. Wages plummeted after the 2008 recession and they have largely failed to recover, resulting in what the Institute for Fiscal Studies (IFS) calls 'a lost decade'[41].

Allowing for inflation, median weekly earnings are still 2% below April 2008 levels – plus there are persistent wage gaps for women and people of colour. Oh, and then there was that worldwide pandemic. So if you're feeling undervalued and burnt out, it's time to at least negotiate what you're worth.

## Are you ready for a pay rise?

If you've worked for your employer for at least a year, have started to go beyond your job description and feel confident you are a good worker, you're in the perfect place to negotiate a pay rise. If you're not sure, take some time to actively find opportunities to shine.

## Pay freeze? Negotiate benefits.

There are many ways to be better compensated for your work. You could ask for a preferable start time, more flexible time off, the option to work from home or a better job title. These can often be easier to negotiate and more valuable to your work–life balance than a small increase in salary.

## Find out what you're worth.

That's right, you absolutely *can* ask your colleagues what they earn. It's the best way to work out if you're being underpaid. If you really can't stomach it, try asking friends in similar roles at other companies and comparing the salaries on career search websites.

## Pick the right time.

Annual pay reviews or performance meetings are the best time to bring up a pay rise – in fact, many managers will be expecting it. But if your company doesn't have regular assessments, ask for a good time to discuss your career with your manager. Let them schedule it at their convenience.

## Craft your business case.

Look carefully at your job description and show how you've gone above and beyond it. Use as much real data as you can. If you can demonstrate things like, say, your project brought in a new client, your new process improved performance or your management style resolved a big problem, that's going to be way easier to talk about than 'I'm really great! I swear!' (I know you really *are* great, but this is capitalism, baby.) Add in positive testimonials from people you work with.

Put all this together in a one-sheet, which you can use as your discussion notes and as a leave-behind. Make sure you write and speak in a positive, confident tone. Remember, you're not some charlatan begging for cash, you're a valued employee proactively demonstrating how you could deliver more.

## Make your desired salary a precise number.

Precise numbers are taken more seriously in negotiations than round ones[42]. So if you've calculated you are worth about £30,000, you'll have a better time negotiating for £31,650. Don't present your salary as a range, either. If you bring £28,000–32,000 to the table, your negotiator will take £28,000 as your lowest acceptable starting point and bargain downwards from there.

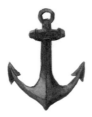

## Ahoy! Weigh anchor!

The first number to be presented in a negotiation is called the anchor. You want your ~~doubloons~~ salary expectations to be the anchor, so be prepared to come straight out with it. Savvy?

## Take some time to decide.

You don't have to agree to an offer on the spot. It's perfectly fine to sleep on it. You may like to come back with a counteroffer.

## Be grateful – even for a rejection.

A salary discussion is a tense and delicate situation. Follow up with genuine thanks for any opportunity to discuss it, regardless of the ultimate outcome. If you no longer want to work for your company, you now have an understandable reason to look for a new position. If you'd rather stay, now's a great time to get clarity on what your employer would need to see before considering a pay rise. If their requirements feel realistic to you, use them as your goals for the coming year. Once you've proved you can do what was asked, you're in the perfect position to negotiate again.

# MOVING UP IN THE PUBLIC SECTOR

Are you a public sector soul? Well, this is as good a place as any for me to thank you for your service. Despite being foundational to our society, it's obvious to me that the work you do is often thankless, over-scrutinised and sometimes even downright dangerous. So *hell yes*, you deserve to be well paid for it. Trouble is, you and I both know that ain't how the public sector works. What you need, my civically minded friend, is a promotion.

## Dress for the job you want.

Look like someone who is ready for the next step. If you wear a uniform, wear it well.

## Update your LinkedIn.

Some organisations do what they call 'virtual shoulder tapping', which means they're out there on LinkedIn actively looking for candidates to promote. So make your shoulder sexy! LinkedIn sexy, of course. Use a bright, professional image, eliminate typos, and try to describe your current role using the skills they'll be looking for in the role you want.

## Get the lay of the land.

Start asking around for feedback from your colleagues and line manager. Unlike the private sector, your manager is not likely to be financially invested in or connected to your success. In other words, they will keep their job regardless of whether or not you do yours well. This can mean they will not be actively looking for ways you could extend and improve yourself – and may even fail to notify you of potential schemes, promotions or opportunities.

So be proactive. Ask your line manager about training, work experience or secondments that serve both your current role and the roles you aspire to. Use your appraisals to discuss skill gaps and set goals to address them. Do some digging on your own, too. Find out how you are perceived, what opportunities are out there, and who's gatekeeping them.

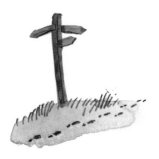

## Project kindness, confidence and adaptability.

Annoyingly, public sector promotions can be less about skill and more about your mindset or certain 'behaviours'. So although it's always important to do your best at work, you can often get more out of being kind, positive, flexible and team-oriented. Don't sweat the small stuff – avoid petty discussions or whingeing at work. Lift your eyes to the horizon and find out what the people above you are dealing with. If you know your one-up's aims, your two-up's intent and your three-up's vision, you'll be able to make your own contribution to their efforts and dramatically improve in their esteem.

## Scope out acceleration schemes and fellowships.

If you can't seem to beat the promotion process, there may be an acceleration scheme, on-the-job training or a fellowship designed to give you those opportunities. The Civil Service, for example, has an entry-level Fast Stream as well as various high-level leadership schemes.

## Get into the habit of networking.

Networking is like manure. (Stay with me.) Spread it evenly across your garden and you get beautiful plants and dazzling flowers. Heap it all in one place and it's just a great big pile of you-know-what. In other words, networking isn't something to do just when you need it.

Grab coffees with people in the area you want to work in. And don't focus solely on high-fliers. You're looking to build real friendships with people close to your level, who in the immediate term will help you do better at your job and in the long term will think of you when an opportunity arises. Some of these networking attempts will come to nothing, but the least that comes of it is a cup of coffee.

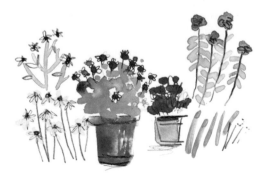

### Find a mentor.

A nice side effect of networking can be that you find a senior colleague who really gets you. Try asking this person if they would consider mentoring you and helping to shape your career. Older colleagues often feel overlooked and unfairly judged by their age, so you may be surprised how many are honoured to be asked to mentor.

### Pick your jobs.

Start scanning internal listings for opportunities. Often these listings have weekly round-up emails you can subscribe to.

### Take advantage of professional development.

Many organisations offer some very decent internal and external continuing professional development (CPD) opportunities, which are a great way to acquire skills, fill in gaps and network.

## Play the game.

Public funding means intense public scrutiny. So be ready to drive yourself slightly mad with paperwork and processes. Try reaching out to colleagues who have already jumped through the hoops – even in different departments – because they can probably share some useful hints and hacks.

The other important aspect to remember is that you will need to somehow prove you are *already* doing the job you want, because public employers tend to ignore potential and use existing behaviours to justify the promotion. Arm yourself with plenty of proof by keeping a journal. Every time you finish a project, solve a problem or resolve a conflict, write it down. Paste in positive testimonials you receive; anything that involves an improvement in statistics is gold dust. Set aside a weekly time to do this as part of your personal development.

# I FEEL UNSUPPORTED. I'M TIRED OF RELYING ON MYSELF

If you're self-employed or working from home, work can quickly feel lonely. One of the hardest things about working on your own is getting stuck and feeling like nobody can help you out in time. Either you're going to solve your problem... or you just aren't. The trick here is to pre-emptively build up a safety net that is ready to catch you when things go all wibbly.

'If your
dream is
only about
you, it's
too small.'

AVA DUVERNAY

## We all stand on the shoulders of giants.

Be wary of idolising people who claim to have achieved ground-breaking success on their own. Because honestly? They're lying. Behind every famous success story there are always foundational elements – like emotional support, a 'small' grant, free workspace, a mentorship, someone cooking the meals or caring for the kids.

Beyond that, every business drives its trucks on our roads, keeps its staff healthy in our NHS and enjoys protection under our law. We're all in this together, so don't feel you should make it alone. Analyse your day-to-day routine and identify areas where you feel you need more help. Perhaps you could be better supported by family and friends, or certain tasks could be outsourced. Give yourself permission to rely on others.

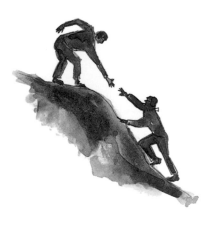

### Cut down on social media.

This sounds counterintuitive, because social media is, well, social, right? Sure, social media is a brilliant way to connect and chat with friends, but it's also a super-great way to feel like everyone else is succeeding without you. I think we all want to project an ideal version of ourselves and it's important to remember that everyone else has bad, lonely, stressful, miserable days, too – they just rarely post about them.

### Remove toxic people.

It's a shame, but there are some people who just don't want your dreams to become reality – especially if you're trying to crack into something cool, creative or entrepreneurial. These people may even be your employees or your clients. It's okay to let yourself drift away from haters and frenemies.

### Find a mentor.

If you're fortunate enough to know someone in a position of power in your industry, see if you can negotiate a formal mentorship with them. If not, there are great professional mentorships available for a fee, such as Script Angel for screenwriters.

## Cultivate a peer network.

There are plenty of people out there who understand exactly what you're trying to do and how hard it can be. It's just a matter of finding them. Connecting with and supporting your peers will be a huge boost to your wellbeing, stamina and sense of place. If you're not sure where to start, try researching your relevant guilds, unions, networks and professional clubs. If you're creative, start sniffing around things like art shows, workshops, poetry slams, zine fairs and film festivals.

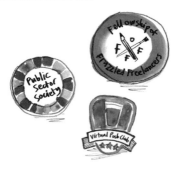

## Find or found a positive-critique group.

This is similar to having a peer network, except with the focus of regularly meeting to exchange and critique work. I found myself in a writer's group after attending a short course on fiction writing. (We were the ones who went to the pub!)

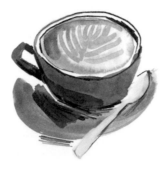

### Book in coffees, dinners and occasions.

As you don't have the luxury of random work gatherings, it's important to be proactive with friends, scheduling in regular times to see them. I'm terrible at this, but always feel so revitalised when I finally do it.

### Try a co-working space.

These can be expensive, but are nonetheless proof that if you're freelance or a remote worker, you don't have to feel lonely or stuck. Some public libraries have an affordable 'rent-a-desk' situation, or you could research residency schemes designed for writers, artists and start-ups.

# I DON'T FEEL VALUED

Your ideas are ignored. Your colleagues forget your name. Nobody seems to think of you when an opportunity comes along. Whether you work for a big faceless corporation or a teensy-weensy start-up, it's easy to feel like a little cog in a huge machine, grinding away on the long road to burnout. But the truth is, we humans are pretty self-absorbed creatures and we don't tend to notice things unless they're screaming at us. So here are some classy ways to, well, scream at your boss.

## Give praise to get praise.

It sounds counterintuitive, but one of the best ways to get more positive reinforcement is to go around giving it to everyone else. If you praise your colleagues, including your boss, most will feel tempted to respond by complimenting something you have done, too. This encourages them to consider you, which can lead them to realise things about you they hadn't noticed.

Celebrating team wins is another easy way to create positive energy. Even if you're brave enough only to send round an email, taking the time to publicly praise others will shine a light on your strengths, too.

## Use 'echoing' in meetings.

Echoing was developed by Obama's female White House staffers to help overcome the unconscious bias against them and their ideas. The way it works is simple: when one woman made a key point in a meeting, another woman would reiterate it immediately afterwards, giving credit to its author. But echoing doesn't have to be Secret Women's Business.

Get together with a friend or a group and arrange to subtly echo each other. Or if you have a big meeting coming up, take the time to win support from an influential attendee by going through your ideas with them beforehand. If they like your ideas they will naturally echo you, helping you fill in the gaps if you stumble in the moment.

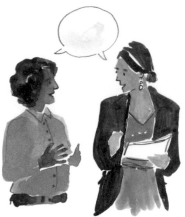

## Build your personal brand.

Branding is a cheesy way to talk about your reputation at work. Trouble is, most of us let others define our brand for us. Yours might be 'the shy one who loathes teamwork' when really you think you are 'the positive one who gets things done'. Take the time to define the phrase you want to pop into people's heads when they think of you. Underneath this, list out all of the personal attributes that support your phrase.

Pay close attention to your interactions with others at work, including via email, and make a conscious effort to apply your brand attributes. If you can, seek feedback from trusted colleagues on how you're coming across. It can take several months of concerted effort to rebrand yourself, but putting yourself in control of your reputation will almost always pay off in the long term.

## Don't apologise for your input.

If you're feeling undervalued, you may unconsciously use timid language when you do speak up. 'This is probably nothing, but...' Don't tell people how to feel about your ideas or suggestions. If you say it's bad, they'll think it's bad. Try to express yourself clearly and let them decide.

## Spill your secrets.

Sometimes, when it feels like your colleagues don't notice you, it's really that they don't know enough about you. A surprisingly effective way to spark or deepen a friendship is to divulge a personal secret[43]. Before you go tarting up that PowerPoint on your top ten sex moves, secrets can be quite little things. Perhaps it's that you're feeling stressed, you've been re-watching *The Wire*, or you're learning to bake croissants.

Talk openly about your hobbies and interests, or signal them in other ways. Change your phone wallpaper, decorate your desk, dress more confidently, bring in that homemade bread. And don't try to professionalise it or turn it into some gambit for the boss's attention. Be authentic and people will value you for it.

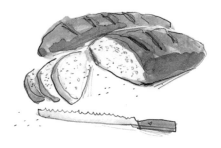

## Build your confidence with gratitude.

Are you ignoring any positive comments and hearing only negatives? Practising gratitude is a proven way to counteract negative feelings, like envy, social comparison and cynicism[44]. The easiest exercise with the most solid research behind it is 'gratitude journaling'[45]. All you need to do is regularly write down a few things that you feel grateful for. They don't have to be big things, or even related to your work. Just nice things that you happened to notice today.

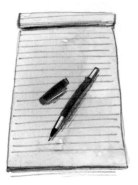

# Gratitude

I have a confession to make: I'm not very good at mindfulness or meditation. It's not that these techniques don't work – they do and for lots of people. They are a great way to put yourself in the moment so you can stop worrying about everything for once. But sometimes that can make me feel like I'm just shoving my head in the sand.

Gratitude is different. It's not about pretending you're okay. It's about paying more attention to and adding equal weight to the things in your life that are okay. And there's actually a lot of science behind it. Gratitude stimulates the pathways in the brain associated with reward[46] and makes it easier to recall positive memories[47]. People who are grateful tend to be happier, less dissatisfied, and suffer less from depression, addiction and burnout[48].

And all it takes is a pen and some paper. Simply spend a few moments writing down the things that you feel grateful for today, whether they're small, silly or serious. I am often extremely grateful for freshly baked croissants.

I find practising gratitude is a great way to take a small break during the day – one that not only gets you away from all the screens but makes you smile.

# MY WORKPLACE FEELS TOXIC

Your boss never leaves the office. You can never conquer your workload. And you're forced to compete with your colleagues in a world where a pat on the back could be a recce for a knife. Yep, you're trapped in a toxic work culture – a real burnout petri dish.

This sort of environment is especially common in 'elite' professional organisations, like consulting and law firms. The idea is that you thrash yourself for a decade or two and 'make partner' in order to finally enjoy some work–life balance. But this evaporated after the 2008 recession, and now even senior employees can't catch a break.

## Success is not the same as working 70 hours a week.

There is nothing heroic about working 1.5 times the legal work week, but many of us have been conditioned to feel pride in overworking. Consider who this mindset benefits. Your company gets a load of extra work for free and manages to normalise exhaustion, making it seem like *you're* the failure when you burn out. And for your trouble? You'll enjoy deteriorated performance, plummeting motivation and an increased risk of stroke[49]. If you regularly work 11-hour days, you're twice as likely to suffer a major depressive episode[50].

Recognise that a culture of overwork is not heroic, successful or healthy. Either you need to accept that you must risk your health and mental wellbeing in order to rise in this organisation, or be prepared to do something about it.

## Notice your triggers.

Recognise when the culture or your colleagues try to manipulate you. Do you feel you should judge others for working fewer hours than you? Are you made to feel worthless for not doing as much as your insecure, overachieving boss? Are you working overtime for a reason? If you must overwork, make sure it's for a specific goal or time period.

## Are you an 'insecure overachiever'?

Laura Empson coined this term in her book *Leading Professionals*, which contains a study of 500 senior professionals across the world[51]. 'Insecure overachievers are exceptionally capable and fiercely ambitious, yet driven by a profound sense of their own inadequacy,' Empson explains. This phenomenon tends to develop in childhood, perhaps owing to financial or physical deprivation, or a belief that parental love depended on behaving and performing well.

In her research, Empson found that professional organisations deliberately recruit insecure overachievers, as they self-motivate and self-discipline. These organisations also make a secret of how each employee is rated, knowing that insecure overachievers will work extra hard just to be safe. Despite this, insecure overachievers believe they are overworking by choice and never hold their organisation or its leaders to account. Nothing changes, and the insecure overachievers who rise to the top unconsciously replicate toxic systems of control and overwork.

If this sounds familiar, it's time to acknowledge the role your organisation plays in your work behaviours. Open up to colleagues you trust – or friends in similar situations – and start dispelling the myth of the invincible professional and the 'choice' to overwork.

### Decide what success means to you.

Don't buy into the idea of constantly competing with and comparing yourself to your colleagues. Decide what a successful day looks like to you and embrace the tunnel vision.

### Celebrate your achievements.

Don't do that thing where as soon as you've achieved something, you tell yourself it was nothing and immediately set your sights on some bigger, brighter achievement. Listen when you are praised, celebrate your successes and learn to take compliments. If you don't develop conscious awareness of the good things, you allow your career to be defined by the bad things.

### Get a life.

Do you have a life outside of work? Unproductive time? Friends? Hobbies? Give yourself more reasons to come home at night.

## Discuss your workplace culture with your team and leadership.

The good news is, it sounds smart to talk about wellness and work–life balance. Most organisations interpret it as a feel-good way to boost productivity, and you can use that cynical angle to get the ball rolling. Pitch yourself as the proactive problem-solver, going above and beyond to help everyone in your company do better and feel better. (If you're young or lower down the ladder, try clubbing in with like-minded allies to get your views tabled.)

Start by suggesting the implementation of wellness programmes, then slowly layer in ideas like transparency of workloads, working from home, mental health discussions, counselling options, and the costs and health risks of overworking. Think of it like turning an oil tanker. It takes ages, but one push at a time will bring the boat around.

# I'M STRUGGLING TO MANAGE OTHERS

Let me guess. You thought that management role was going to grow your career with a nice little pay bump. What you actually found was an unending doom-spiral of bureaucracy, whip-cracking and emotional labour. Your team don't want to be managed, but you're accountable for their output. Your boss wants endless improvements, but has no idea how or why. Your days have become fraught, frustrating and exhausting – and everyone thinks *you're* the bad guy! Welcome to management hell. It's time to bust you out before you burn out.

'You must
not lose faith
in humanity.
Humanity is an
ocean; if a few
drops of the
ocean are dirty,
the ocean does
not become dirty.'

**GANDHI**

## Management is the main job.

One survey of 150 leaders found nearly two-thirds don't actually like managing[52]. The most common story is being promoted out of the 'real job' and feeling frustrated about now spending all day doing 'management stuff'. But the thing is, *we choose our jobs*. So be honest with yourself. Despite the compromises, do you still like your job enough to spend all of your day doing it? If you don't, that's fine! But it may be worth skipping to page 177 to think about whether this is the job for you.

## Your style is the best style.

There are certain stereotypes we tend to associate with managers – talking tough, using acronyms, David Brent, Gordon Gekko. But if you're trying too hard to use a management style that doesn't suit your personality, when you do struggle you'll only feel more and more convinced you're not cut out for it. The trick is to develop a management style that comes from who you really are, which you can subtly adapt to motivate the different personalities on your team. Field Marshal Slim defined leadership as 'just plain you'. If you're authentic, people will be more likely to trust you.

## Open communication channels.

Your people are often your biggest problem and your most obvious solution. Opening clear lines of communication and creating an environment where everyone feels comfortable sharing is the best way to restore transparency, accountability and trust. A great baseline is morning work-in-progress meetings (WIPs), where everyone shares where they're at and any problems they're facing. From there, add in optional ways for your team to reach out, including emails, one-to-ones and strolling around the workplace.

It's worth bearing in mind that the problems people bring you often seem like they have nothing to do with their job. But behind every piece of work that gets delivered is a complicated person with their own battles. Don't panic – it's not your job to solve these problems. All you need to do is actively listen and help them feel supported. People will often tell you what they need.

## Be the older sibling, not a best mate.

As much as you'd like to be everyone's friend, you have a position of authority. Be clear about what is expected of your team and stick to it, rather than bending the rules or dragging everyone down the pub because you're the nice boss. If you can maintain clarity and fairness in what you do, your team will like you anyway.

## Don't assume people understand your logic.

When you need to inform someone of something – especially if it is a big change or bad news – the most important part is explaining why. Because if you don't explain your reasons, people will come up with their own. It is often better to be tactfully honest about how a decision was reached rather than sugar-coat it in corporate language. Letting others in on your process helps them feel part of it, and not as though they are being forced to swallow a bitter pill.

## Don't just demand success. Create the conditions for it.

Modern work is going through a bit of a tussle between management and coaching. Management tends to be about telling, directing and specific outcomes. Coaching, meanwhile, is about exploring, facilitating, long-term improvement and many possible outcomes. Some situations really do require strict management, but for the most part, people increasingly prefer being coached. The good news is, coaching is a much healthier workload for you. Relieve yourself of the pressure of always knowing what to do, and instead focus on empowering your team to make their own judgements and set their own benchmarks.

## See the art in what everyone does.

Put bluntly, never piss off the cook. No matter how simple a job seems, don't scrimp on the appreciation and feedback. Everyone needs to feel like what they are doing is important. Don't jump straight to talking about what's wrong with the work, even if it's glaringly obvious to you. Acknowledge what is working before you move on to what isn't, or your team member will hear nothing but failure and they could spiral into a negative feedback loop.

## Is your team having an identity crisis?

Most companies spend a decent wedge developing a corporate identity – the concept, language and visuals used to communicate their brand to others. Corporate IDs are usually dense documents full of things like pillars and values and sales pitches, and they're considered so vital, they are redefined every few years. So why is it so rare to do this internally? What use is defining a brand to others if we can't explain why we're here to ourselves?

Being in a management position is a brilliant opportunity to build a fulfilling purpose and culture. It doesn't matter if you don't know exactly what would work. What's important is an interrogative mindset that starts with you and actively involves your entire team. Who are we? Why are we here? What kind of people do we want to be? How should we treat each other? What kind of place do we want to work in? What's our culture? How can we be good ancestors?

You may find that some responses to these questions contradict what your company wants. Perhaps you all agree you want a family atmosphere, but your company provokes competitive behaviours by ranking employees based on results. These are conflicts of interest that are probably root causes of dissatisfaction, which may require serious interventions to resolve. Be brave. Fight for your team if you have to.

## Beware management fads.

In America in the 1890s, Frederick Taylor invented a 'scientific method for efficiency'. He published papers with fudged numbers, claiming he had quadrupled output at Bethlehem Steel. Today we know he was a complete fraud, but Taylor's work nevertheless spawned the industry of 'management science', directly inspiring systems like Six Sigma, the Toyota Production System, Lean Start-up and Agile.

These systems 'use the metaphor of the organisation as a kind of machine, a computer that can be reprogrammed, rebooted, and updated with new business processes,' says Dan Lyons, in his book *Lab Rats: Why Modern Work Makes People Miserable*. 'It's easy to laugh at Agile and write it all off as another nutty fad, except that in some places this is really causing harm. The original version of Taylorism ... drove men to physical exhaustion and injury. Modern-day Taylorism takes an even bigger toll but on the psyche.'

Instead, Lyons advocates what University of Portsmouth researcher Sally Rumbles calls 'the no-shit-Sherlock school of management'. What really works boils down to treating people how you would like to be treated, and building trust, pride and camaraderie.

# I FEEL JEALOUS OF OTHERS AND THEIR SUCCESS

When you want a particular success very badly, it can feel like anyone who comes close to it is 'in your way'. But the truth is almost the opposite. It means you believe you cannot have that success. So give yourself some perspective. A lot of modern organisations are hard-wired to make you compete against your colleagues – and worse, will make it difficult or even dangerous to chat openly about work–life balance, making you feel like the only one struggling with it.

### Nobody is actually competing with you.

There is not a finite amount of success in the world. Someone else's success is not your failure. Your career is not a zero-sum game. In fact, the more you embrace and amplify the success of your peers, the more you will find opportunities radiated back at you.

'We are what we pretend to be, so we must be careful what we pretend to be.'

KURT VONNEGUT

## There's no mathematical formula for success.

Frankly, if there was, I'd be writing that book. So if you find yourself envying other people's success and thinking, 'But, why?! I've worked just as hard as them!' it's time to stop measuring your apples against their oranges. We're all on unique journeys, with myriad different skills, attitudes, opportunities, connections and, of course, luck.

## Find a collective. Start a movement.

One of the best ways to feel that your success is building momentum is to club in with like-minded souls. Maybe you're all trying to become brain surgeons. Maybe you're all trying to publish a novel. Maybe you just like each other's management style. Think about all the famous collectives over the years – The Socrates School, The Bloomsbury Set, The Factory. Maybe yours will be the next big thing.

## Stop evaluating your career by social media.

One of the most addictive elements of social media is the identity affirmation. Whether it's the glossy filtered photography of Instagram or the overhyped corporate jargon of LinkedIn, these are places that allow you to curate an idealised version of yourself for the world to admire.

If you're feeling down about yourself, the problems here are twofold: one, you're fooling yourself with a false exaggeration of your success. And two, you're being fooled by the apparent success of those you follow. Social media can be important to your career, but you get to decide how and when you use it.

If you can't handle the idea of a detox, avoid online activities that make you feel worse. Focus on following a positive community of people who reflect what you are trying to do. (Translation: follow more cats, fewer prats.)

## Are you flitting between unfinished projects?

Do you have problems with follow-through? Are you really putting in the time? Try to identify where you are failing to finish and why. Maybe you need to raise more funds. Maybe you need to better manage your health. The answer is not likely to be fun or simple, but being honest with yourself and your work habits will always help.

## Do you have a plan?

I don't mean a dream collage; I mean a bona fide business or career plan. According to Bloomberg, fully 80% of new businesses fail in less than two years – most owing to having no plan, a lack of cash or a poor value proposition[53]. (A value proposition is a clear 'why go with me' statement.) Although a career or business plan will vary dramatically depending on your particular industry, taking the time to craft a serious strategy will dramatically increase your odds of success.

## Go talk to the people who make you jealous.

I'm serious. Unless you're obsessed with an extremely famous person who would probably hit you with a restraining order, go and find out what your peers are doing so right. You might even become friends.

# I WAS HIRED WITH PROMISES THAT NEVER MATERIALISE

Ah, those halcyon days of starting a new job! Everyone seems so positive. There are going to be office parties, benefits and bonuses. And if you work really hard, you'll get promoted by the end of the year!... and nothing happens. Ever. Then you steam through all five stages of grief and wake up fully burnt out. Well, hold on. Let's see if there's anything we can do about it.

### Consider any wider changes.

Has there been a massive restructure? New leadership? Pay freeze? A wave of redundancies? It may be that the context in which your promise was made has completely disappeared. Determine whether your promiser is being honest with you or just stringing you along.

### Listen to actions, not words.

If you've done your part but what you've been promised has been continually deferred over a long period of time, accept that it's not coming. You cannot trust this person. It is now time to move on or do something about it.

### Have you mentioned it lately?

Work-related promises seem to fall alongside money, politics and religion: it feels rude to talk openly about them at work. But if you have been promised something and you've never brought it up again – especially if it was more than a year ago – your promiser has either forgotten, thinks that *you* have forgotten, or worse, thinks that you don't mind. Start by casually bringing it up in a private conversation to gauge their reaction.

### Can you get the ball rolling yourself?

If you were promised things like company social events, certain equipment or access to training, it's generally better to start things off yourself rather than reminding someone they have let you down. Research what it would take to fulfil what you've been promised and present this with a proactive energy. You'll be surprised how easily things happen once someone takes charge – and how positively it reflects on you for doing it.

## Formally raise your concerns.

If you were promised something serious, like a promotion, and your hints and proactive measures aren't getting you anywhere, it's time to have a talk. Schedule a meeting to discuss your career with the person who made the promise. Lay down the facts of the situation as you understood them. Try your best to be calm and unemotional, making it more about your eagerness than their broken promise.

## Try again somewhere else.

If you can't get anywhere in your current role, you need to accept that your employer is a carrot dangler. Start looking for another job. If you do receive a job offer and you still like your original company, you may be able to use the offer to prove you are worth the unfulfilled promise. If that doesn't work, move on, and try to get any further promises in writing.

# I'M NOT SURE I WANT THIS CAREER ANY MORE

This really is the ultimate question. If you have been managing your health, your emotions, your expectations, your finances, your career plan and everything in between, and you still feel burnt out, you may begin to wonder if this is all worth it. You might just be in a rough patch. Or you might be realising this isn't for you.

### Can you take the good with the bad?

On some level, all jobs suck. The trick is finding the type of suck you can put up with. For me, freelance writing is often poorly paid, high stress and full of harsh feedback – but it also lets me express myself, build a creative body of work and run my own career. Do the pros outweigh the cons for you? Make a list and see.

## If it was easy, everyone would do it.

Don't feel bad that you're struggling. We're all struggling. (Honestly! Even the people at the top of their game have days that are total crap.) So if you're not in a good place but still don't want to quit, take all the time you need to rediscover the love. You're going to need it at the top.

## You are not a failure for changing your mind.

There was no way to know what your job was going to be like until you tried it. And you really tried it! There's no reason to regret doing your best. In fact, leaving a job you no longer enjoy is a sign of emotional maturity. Moving forward, you will have equipped yourself with all kinds of skills, contacts and knowledge that will help you define your next move. Lots of successful people make huge career changes later on in their lives.

## Interrogate yourself.

One technique is to imagine all the things you would choose to do if you had infinite lives. Another is to notice the things you tend to do when you finally have some free time. A third strategy is to imagine who you want to be at 50 and work backwards, discovering the steps it would take to get there.

If you are still struggling to ask yourself the right questions that lead to your purpose in life, it can be helpful to talk to close friends and family. Sit down together with some blank paper and coloured markers and let your mind free-associate the things that you think make a good life. There are no wrong answers.

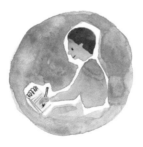

## Evaluate your life and your dreams.

Unfortunately, this is one of those things that nobody can truly help you with, but for what it's worth, I've found the Japanese concept of ikigai very useful. Ikigai roughly translates as purpose in life or raison d'être.

As you can see in the diagram to the right, ikigai is a sort of Venn diagram with four primary elements:

- What you love
- What the world needs
- What you are good at
- What you can be paid for

The idea is to try to move away from what's 'right' – things like good grades, good earnings, high prestige – and move towards what's right for you. Your ikigai will not usually be something grand or extraordinary, but more of a sustainable passion that will carry you through your whole life. The American architect, inventor and author Buckminster Fuller worked his way through a deep depression by asking himself: 'What is my job on the planet? What is it that needs doing, that I know something about, that probably won't happen unless I take responsibility for it?'

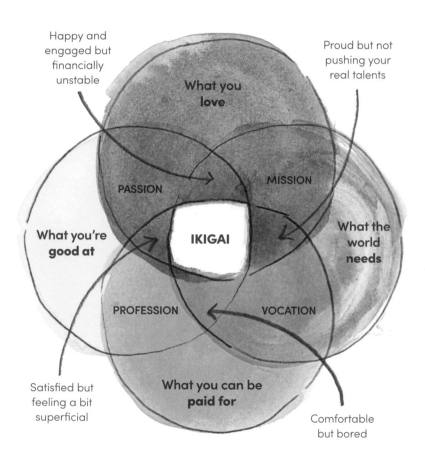

Happy and engaged but financially unstable

Proud but not pushing your real talents

What you **love**

PASSION

MISSION

What you're **good at**

IKIGAI

What the world **needs**

PROFESSION

VOCATION

Satisfied but feeling a bit superficial

What you can be **paid for**

Comfortable but bored

## I chose a career because of money, prestige or my parents.

It can be horrifying to feel like you rolled along on the 'right' tracks only to arrive at the 'wrong' destination. You did everything that was expected of you – got the grades, got the job, got the promotions – except you somehow forgot to listen to your heart. Realising you want a career change tends to bring up fears around money, status and age. You're 'too old', you 'missed' your chances, and besides, who is going to pay for your dog's alopecia medication? Cut the crap. If you were smart enough to get where you are, you'll be able to continue your lifestyle in a job you actually enjoy.

The first thing to do is stop thinking of a career change as some whiplash-inducing U-turn and start thinking of it like changing lanes. You probably have a lot of transferable skills, as well as a strong idea of what you like and don't like, what you're good at and not good at. You also will have a solid starting point for networking. Friends have friends. Look for interesting people, not jobs, and you'll start to get a much better idea of what you'd like to do and who with. From there, you can dip your toe in with a side project or an evening course. Before you know it you'll be hitting the indicator and gliding into your new spot.

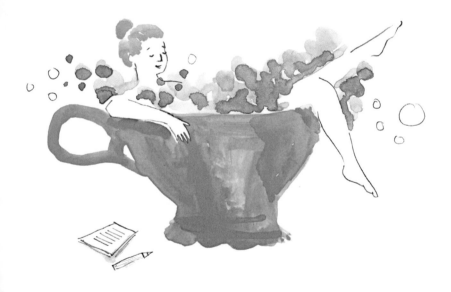

# READING LIST

While researching this book, I found myself repeatedly turning to the work of these brilliant people. Some are funny, some are serious, all are brutally honest.

Laura Empson, *Leading Professionals: Power, Politics, and Prima Donnas* (Oxford University Press: Oxford, 2017).

Aaron Gillies, *How to Survive the End of the World (When It's In Your Own Head)* (Two Roads: London, 2018).

Matt Haig, *Reasons to Stay Alive* (Canongate: London, 2015).

James Kerr, *Legacy: What the All Blacks Can Teach Us About the Business of Life* (Constable: London, 2013).

Dan Lyons, *Lab Rats: Why Modern Work Makes People Miserable* (Atlantic Books: London, 2019).

Jenny Odell, *How to Do Nothing: Resisting the Attention Economy* (Melville House: New York, 2019).

Dennis Palumbo, *Writing from the Inside Out: Transforming Your Psychological Blocks to Release the Writer Within* (Wiley: New York, 2000).

Shonda Rhimes, *Year of Yes: How to Dance It Out, Stand In the Sun and Be Your Own Person* (Simon & Schuster: London, 2016).

Zeynep Ton, *The Good Jobs Strategy: How the Smartest Companies Invest in Employees to Lower Costs and Boost Profits* (New Harvest: New York, 2014).

# ENDNOTES

1. Saul Gilbert, 'Thermoregulation as a Sleep Signalling System', *Sleep Medicine Reviews* 8, no. 2 (April 2004): 81–93.

2. T.A. LeGates, 'Light as a Central Modulator of Circadian Rhythms, Sleep and Affect', *Nature Reviews Neuroscience* 15, no. 7 (July 2014): 443–54.

3. Madhumita Murgia, 'How Stress Affects Your Brain', TED-Ed Online, November 2015. Video, 4:01: https://www.ted.com/talks/madhumita_murgia_how_stress_affects_your_brain

4. Suzanne Segerstrom and Gregory Miller, 'Psychological Stress and the Human Immune System: A Meta-Analytic Study of 30 Years of Inquiry', *Psychological Bulletin* 130, no. 4 (2004): 601–630.

5. Health and Safety Executive, 'Health and Safety at Work: Summary Statistics for Great Britain 2019' (2019): https://www.hse.gov.uk/statistics/overall/hssh1819.pdf

6. Kevin Yackle, et al, 'Breathing control center neurons that promote arousal in mice', *Science* 31, no. 6332 (March 2017): 1411–1415.

7. Kostandin Kushlev and Elizabeth Dunn, 'Checking email less frequently reduces stress', *Computers in Human Behavior* 43 (February 2015): 220–228.

8. University of Edinburgh, 'More Facebook friends means more stress, says report', *ScienceDaily*: www.sciencedaily.com/releases/2012/11/121126131218.htm (accessed 9 May 2020).

9. Andrew Steptoe, et al, 'Social isolation, loneliness, and all-cause mortality in older men and women', *PNAS* 110, no.15 (April 2013): 5797–5801.

10.   Oscar Ybarra, et al, 'Friends (And Sometimes Enemies) With Cognitive Benefits: What Types of Social Interactions Boost Executive Functioning?' *Social Psychological and Personality Science* 2, no. 3 (2011): 253–261.

11.   Harry Reis, et al, 'Familiarity does indeed promote attraction in live interaction', *Journal of Personality and Social Psychology* 101, no. 3 (September 2011): 557–570.

12.   Erica Jackson, 'STRESS RELIEF: The role of exercise in stress management', *ACSM's Health & Fitness Journal* 17, no. 3 (May/June 2013): 14–19.

13.   Matthew Stults-Kolehmainen and Rajita Sinha, 'The Effects of Stress on Physical Activity and Exercise', *Sports Medicine* 44 (2014): 81–121.

14.   James Kerr, *Legacy: What the All Blacks Can Teach Us About the Business of Life* (London: Constable, 2013).

15.   Libby Sander, 'The Case for Finally Cleaning your Desk', *Harvard Business Review* (25 March 2019): https://hbr.org/2019/03/the-case-for-finally-cleaning-your-desk

16.   Joshua Rubenstein, David Meyer and Jeffrey Evans, 'Executive Control of Cognitive Processes in Task Switching', *Journal of Experimental Psychology: Human Perception and Performance* 27, no. 24 (2001): 763–797. https://www.apa.org/pubs/journals/releases/xhp274763.pdf

17.   Sofie Bates, 'A decade of data reveals that heavy multitaskers have reduced memory, Stanford psychologist says', *Stanford News* (25 October 2018): https://news.stanford.edu/2018/10/25/decade-data-reveals-heavy-multitaskers-reduced-memory-psychologist-says/

18.   John Robinson, et al, 'The Overestimated Workweek Revisited', *U.S. Bureau of Labor Statistics, Monthly Labor Review* (June 2011): 43–53. https://www.bls.gov/opub/mlr/2011/06/art3full.pdf

19. Akiyo Sasaki-Otomaru, et al, 'Effect of Regular Gum Chewing on Levels of Anxiety, Mood, and Fatigue in Healthy Young Adults', *Clinical Practice & Epidemiology in Mental Health* 7 (2011): 133–139.

20. Dennis Palumbo, *Writing from the Inside Out: Transforming Your Psychological Blocks to Release the Writer Within* (Wiley: New York, 2000).

21. Shonda Rhimes, *Year of Yes: How to Dance It Out, Stand In the Sun and Be Your Own Person* (Simon & Schuster: UK, 2016).

22. Reis, et al (2011).

23. Mark Goulston, *Talking to Crazy: How to Deal with the Irrational and Impossible People in Your Life* (Amacom: Calfornia, 2015).

24. Richard Pulsford, et al, 'Associations of sitting behaviours with all-cause mortality over a 16-year follow-up: The Whitehall II study', *International Journal of Epidemiology* 44, no. 6 (December 2015): 1909–1916.

25. BUPA, 'Working from home can be a pain in the neck' (19 May 2017): www.bupa.co.uk/newsroom/ourviews/working-from-home-can-be-a-pain-in-the-neck

26. Mohamed Boubekri and Ivy Cheung, et al, 'Impact of workplace daylight exposure on sleep, physical activity, and quality of life', *Journal of Clinical Sleep Medicine* 10, no. 6 (June 2014): 603–611.

27. British Chiropractic Association, 'Working from Home: Back Health Risk' (12 April 2016): chiropractic-uk.co.uk/uk-risk-back-health-when-working-from-home

28. Harvard Medical School, 'Blue light has a dark side: Exposure to blue light at night, emitted by electronics and energy-efficient lightbulbs, can be harmful to your health', *Harvard Health Publishing* (13 August 2018): www.health.harvard.edu/staying-healthy/blue-light-has-a-dark-side

29. Jessica Schmerler, 'Why Is Blue Light before Bedtime Bad for Sleep?', *Scientific American* (1 September 2015): www.scientificamerican.com/article/q-a-why-is-blue-light-before-bedtime-bad-for-sleep

30. James Dillon, Lei Zheng, et al, 'Transmission of Light to the Aging Human Retina: Possible Implication for Age Related Macular Degeneration', *Experimental Eye Research* 79, no. 6 (December 2004): 653–9.

31. O.C. Tanner Institute, '2020 Global Culture Report' (2019): https://www.octanner.com/content/dam/oc-tanner/documents/white-papers/2019/INT-GCR2020-12.pdf

32. Andrea Leaman and Bill Bordass, 'Productivity in buildings: the "killer" variables', *Building Research & Information* 27, no. 1 (1997): 4–19.

33. Rachel Morrison and Keith Macky, 'The demands and resources arising from shared office spaces', *Applied Ergonomics* 60 (April 2017): 103–115.

34. Joseph Allen, et al, 'Associations of Cognitive Function Scores with Carbon Dioxide, Ventilation, and Volatile Organic Compound Exposures in Office Workers: A Controlled Exposure Study of Green and Conventional Office Environments', *Environmental Health Perspectives* 124, no. 6 (June 2016): 805–812.

35. Simon Banbury and Dianne Berry, 'Disruption of office-related tasks by speech and office noise', *British Journal of Psychology* 89, no. 3 (August 1998): 499–517.

36. O.C. Tanner Institute, 'Performance Accelerated: A New Benchmark for Initiating Employee Engagement, Retention and Results' (June 2011): https://www.octanner.com/content/dam/oc-tanner/documents/global-research/White_Paper_Performance_Accelerated.pdf

37. Audrey Bergouignan, et al, 'Effect of frequent interruptions of prolonged sitting on self-perceived levels of energy, mood, food cravings and cognitive function', *International Journal of Behavioral Nutrition and Physical Activity* 13, 113 (2016).

38. Zeynep Ton, *The Good Jobs Strategy: How the Smartest Companies Invest in Employees to Lower Costs and Boost Profits* (New Harvest: New York, 2014).

39. Market Finance, 'UK SMEs Stretched Further by Late Payments', *Market Finance: In The Press* (9 December 2019): https://blog.marketfinance.com/2019/12/09/uk-smes-stretched-further-by-late-payments/

40. Amanda Palmer, *The Art of Asking: How I Learned to Stop Worrying and Let People Help* (Piatkus: London, 2014).

41. Jonathan Cribb and Paul Johnston, 'Employees' Earnings Since the Great Recession: The Latest Picture', *Institute for Fiscal Studies* (29 October 2019): https://www.ifs.org.uk/publications/14530

42. Malia Mason, et al, 'Precise offers are potent anchors: Conciliatory counteroffers and attributions of knowledge in negotiations', *Journal of Experimental and Social Psychology* 49, no. 4 (July 2013): 759–763.

43. Arthur Aron, Elaine Aron, et al, 'The Experimental Generation of Interpersonal Closeness: A Procedure and Some Preliminary Findings', *Personality and Social Psychology* 23, no. 4 (1997): 363–376.

44. Rebecca Solom, Philip Watkins, et al, 'Thieves of Thankfulness: Traits that inhibit gratitude', *Journal of Positive Psychology* 12, no. 2 (April 2016): 120–129.

45. Summer Allen, *The Science of Gratitude* (UC Berkeley: 2018). https://ggsc.berkeley.edu/images/uploads/GGSC-JTF_White_Paper-Gratitude-FINAL.pdf

46. Andrea Caputo, 'The Relationship Between Gratitude and Loneliness: The Potential Benefits of Gratitude for Promoting Social Bonds', *Europe's Journal of Psychology* 11, no. 2 (May 2015): 323–334.

47.  Philip C. Watkins, Jens Uhder & Stan Pichinevskiy, 'Grateful recounting enhances subjective well-being: The importance of grateful processing', *The Journal of Positive Psychology* 10, no. 2 (June 2014): 91–98.

48.  Allen (2018).

49.  Mika Kivimäki, et al, 'Long working hours and risk of coronary heart disease and stroke: a systematic review and meta-analysis of published and unpublished data', *The Lancet* 386, no. 10005 (August 2015): 1739–1746.

50.  Marianna Virtanen, et al, 'Overtime Work as a Predictor of Major Depressive Episode: A 5-Year Follow-Up of the Whitehall II Study', *PLOS ONE* 7, no. 1 (January 2012): 1–5.

51.  Laura Empson, *Leading Professionals: Power, Politics, and Prima Donnas* (Oxford University Press: Oxford, 2017).

52.  Devora Zack, *Managing For People Who Hate Managing: Be a Success by Being Yourself* (Berrett-Koehler Publishers: Oakland, 2012).

53.  Karen Klein, 'The Bottom Line on Startup Failures', *Bloomberg Business* (4 March 2002): www.bloomberg.com/news/articles/2002-03-03/the-bottom-line-on-startup-failures

# You
# got
# this.

Burnout often feels like your fault. You couldn't take the heat and you got smoked. But take a good sniff – that smoke is everywhere. Burnout is great big invisible wildfire, raging through almost every modern workplace, and here we are trying to fight it on our own with cups of tea. So if you take anything from this book, I hope it's this:

**You didn't start the fire.**

**You're not fighting it alone.**

**Things will improve if you take it seriously.**

Let's shake off the blame. Let's chat openly about burnout. And let's hold our workplaces to account.

**May the frost be with you.**